CANCER AND
YOUR PET

CANCER AND YOUR PET

A Guide to Alternative and Integrated Treatment

Marie Cargill

ROWMAN & LITTLEFIELD
Lanham • Boulder • New York • Toronto • Plymouth, UK

Published by Rowman & Littlefield
4501 Forbes Boulevard, Suite 200, Lanham, Maryland 20706
www.rowman.com

10 Thornbury Road, Plymouth PL6 7PP, United Kingdom

British Library Cataloguing in Publication Information Available

Library of Congress Cataloging-in-Publication Data
Cargill, Marie.
  Cancer and your pet : a guide to alternative and integrated treatment /
Marie Cargill.
     pages cm
  Includes bibliographical references and index.
  ISBN 978-1-4422-3029-3 (cloth : alk. paper) — ISBN 978-1-4422-3030-9
(electronic : alk. paper) 1. Veterinary oncology. 2. Pets—Diseases.
3. Cancer in animals. I. Title.
  SF910.T8C37 2014
  636.089'6994—dc23   2013049488

Printed in the United States of America

DEDICATED TO BOTH MY LOVES:
ANIMALS AND ALTERNATIVE MEDICINE

There is one thing stronger than all the armies of the world, and that is an idea whose time has come.

—Victor Hugo

CONTENTS

ACKNOWLEDGMENTS

My sincere appreciation of all the help and encouragement from so many people. There is no way to thank the clients and patients, human and animal, whose support is on every page. I hope they realize they are part of the solution to the best medicine and cancer treatment in particular that they can provide for their pets. My profound gratitude pours out to those who have made the leap of faith to alternative medicine and allowed me to work with their loved pets.

Plus, there are some particular individuals who have made this book possible. Tim Thompson and his computer skills, Dr. Eugene Bernstein and his research help, Bill Graelish for hunting down the research of certain parts of this work, Rachel Cann for her criticism and Jennifer Sacks for her editing, Dr. Marge McMillan for her insights into difficult cases and filling in my blanks on veterinary care, and Sue Farlow, Donna Wood, and Nancy Rosenberg, colleagues in the field of pet care who shared experience and their unique skills.

And to a great agent, Grace Freedson, thanks for believing in the book. Humble gratitude to Kwan Yin.

Above all, I stand in awe of the medicine I practice.

INTRODUCTION

Officially, the six-year-old golden retriever was not a police officer, but to the veterinary staff who were always thrilled to see him, he was "Officer Joey." Joey was a police dog specializing in the detection of narcotics. He was also a cancer survivor. Joey's story is a tribute not only to the integration of varied medical approaches, but also to a brave dog and his determined human family.

Since childhood, Adam—the human most attached to Joey—had had two loves: police work and dogs. It seemed inevitable that he would find a way to put them together. When he grew up, Adam became a police officer. Choosing Joey as a puppy, he immediately started to train the dog for detective work. Joey embarked on his professional career at six months old, and, except for the months when his cancer was being diagnosed and treated, he worked continuously uncovering stashes of heroin, cocaine, and marijuana throughout the state of Massachusetts.

To become a police dog, Joey had to go through 10 weeks of drug academy training with Adam. Early on, Joey learned how to handle a retrieve—a rolled-up towel tossed into a field. He mastered the exercise, starting in a broad outer circle and gradually working inward until he located the retrieve.

The next step involved introducing a drug odor into the towel; the dog learned to associate the odor with his towel. (In police dog training, the animal is never exposed to actual drugs.) As the odor of one drug was mastered, another was added until Joey could recognize the scents of the major drugs he would eventually pursue. Fully trained, Joey, like all narcotic-detecting dogs, could search out hiding places in buildings, vehicles, and boats—anywhere a package could be hidden. When he smelled drugs, the dog would alert his human partner by scratching or biting at the hiding place.

After the initial training, Joey and Adam went through a certification process that qualified them to be put on the local drug task force's on-call list for search-and-raid missions. As a team, the two alone performed 35 school searches in a busy year.

One day Adam noticed a lump on Joey's left wrist area. Two days later, it had tripled in size. Adam took Joey to a veterinarian who misdiagnosed the problem, so when the leg swelled, felt hot to the touch, and couldn't bear weight, Adam made an appointment at a major veterinary teaching hospital. The diagnosis was nerve sheath tumor. A letter Joey's family sent out to 30 clinics and hospitals in the greater Boston area explains the outcome:

To Whom It May Concern,

We are writing you this letter in hope that you may be able to help us. In early March of this year, our three-year-old golden retriever, Joey, was diagnosed with a nerve sheath tumor on the top of his left front paw. He was operated on at a university hospital, shortly after to remove as much of the tumor as possible. Within a month, a lump had reappeared in the same spot, so we began radiation and chemotherapy treatments. Joey went through a series of 17 radiation treatments and also received four doses of a cancer drug. It has been approximately two months since Joey's last treatment, and he still has severe radiation burns. When we brought our concerns to the veterinarians at the university hospital, they had no idea what was causing such bad burns. We went for a second opinion at another animal hospital in Boston. They believed the margins on the radiation machine were too wide, causing permanent damage to his lymph nodes. Since our last visit to the veterinary hospital, we have seen doctors, surgeons, plastic surgeons, and radiologists. They all have varied answers. Short of amputation, they have no ideas what to do. A few suggested skin grafts but at the same time didn't believe they will attach because so much damage has been done. At this point we will try anything. Before we started treatment, Joey was a very active dog. He is also employed by the . . . police department as a narcotics dog. Even though Joey is a work dog, he is foremost a member of our family. We write this letter in hope that someone, somewhere has heard of this before and may be able to offer a suggestion. As I said before, we are willing to try anything.

Adam and Jenny

The letter arrived at the clinic I worked at as a consultant, and the chief veterinarian shared it with me. When Joey came for his first visit with us, nearly three months after completing surgery, radiation, and chemotherapy, he was a very sick dog. He had no appetite, had lost a significant amount of weight, and was experiencing continuous diarrhea. He couldn't put any weight on his bad leg. Joey wore a cone collar over his head to prevent him from getting at the wound, which was very tender and painful to the touch; it oozed and bled. At the hospital, Joey had been put on steroids but suffered a bad reaction to the drug and was then prescribed an antihistamine. The family was facing the possibility that Joey would lose his leg.

For a working animal, amputation means retirement. In Joey's case, it would also mean the loss of all the hours and considerable expense of his training, along with the thousands of dollars Adam and Joey could earn on paying jobs. But Adam's concerns were not primarily financial. If Joey lost his leg, Adam lost a partner.

On Joey's first visit to the clinic, my team and I suggested a treatment plan. Joey would come to the clinic weekly for a series of 10 acupuncture treatments. He would wear a wrap of herbal medicine around his wound at all times and would have to be given an herbal formula in a pill form twice a day. The goal was to use acupuncture for pain relief and to rejoin the nerve innervation between the leg and the paw. The herbal wrap would keep the wound granulating—forming new, living tissue and blood supply. The herbal formula taken internally would revitalize Joey's appetite, stop the diarrhea, and help him regain his stamina. Later, when the leg was healed, the herbal formula would be changed to one that would revitalize his immune system and help it destroy any residual cancer cells.

The family reported that Joey ate three cans of food the night after his first treatment and was continuing to eat at a hearty pace after that. As instructed, either Adam or Jenny brought Joey into the clinic to have his wrap changed every day for a week, then less frequently as the treatment continued. Joey seemed to be in much less pain; he started to put weight on the injured leg. He became more energetic and alert, and the diarrhea was gone. The wound shrank to 2.2 centimeters in one month. The wraps, acupuncture treatments, and herbal medicines were working well, and there was no evidence of tumor recurrence or infection.

At this point, Adam received a call from one of the hospitals to which he and Jenny had sent their letter. An appointment had been made for Joey to be examined by a team of practitioners there.

As Joey entered the exam area, the team leader stared at the dog and then at Adam. He seemed annoyed. Adam told me later that this dog did not look at all like the picture that had gone out with the letter. Adam explained that since the letter had been sent, Joey had been undergoing a program of treatment; what the physicians and other practitioners were seeing was the result of the program. It turned out that no one in the group had heard of treatment through wraps and herbal medicines. They were cognizant of acupuncture but nevertheless could not understand how it had reestablished circulation in the leg.

Adam allowed the physicians, radiologists, nurses, and other staff members to examine Joey, but since Joey was doing so well, Adam did not accept any advice or treatment suggestions from them. The visit had little effect on Joey's therapy plan; whether or not it had any impact on the team members we will never know.

Over the following weeks, Joey's wound healed, and the tissue hardened. He was eating—absorbing the nutrients in his food and gaining weight—and using his leg. There was no more pain, no more diarrhea, no more weakness, and, we hoped, no more cancer. When weekly visits were no longer needed, the plan moved into a new phase. Adam brought Joey in for acupuncture four to six times throughout the following year as a preventive measure, and he continued getting his herbal medicine to benefit his immune system.

Four months after his initial visit to the clinic, Officer Joey was back at work. He had regained weight, energy, his appetite, and full mobility. Because so much time had elapsed since his medical treatment began, he and Adam went back to school for recertification. Joey performed well and passed all his tests. He and Adam would continue working as a team for several years to come.

Many of us owe our lives and limbs—and our pets' lives and limbs—to modern technological medical intervention. While these advances should be celebrated, it would be foolhardy for us to look to modern technology as the only means to treat illness. Cases such as Joey's show how enlarging the scope of treatment by adding alternative medicines—therapies that currently lie outside mainstream Western practice—can make the curing process much more effective than the standard one-size-fits-all approaches offered by conventional medicine. Since much of cancer work requires highly technical expertise, strategies that incorporate nutrition, supplements, herbs, and other therapies for their powerful anticancer effects also empower you to play a much greater role in helping your pet to heal.

Cancer is both a chronic and a systemic illness. The limited survival rate does not result from lack of trying but rather emerges from the very simplistic model that modern medicine uses. The modern model sees a tumor as an alien thing that must be killed. But to believe that the tumor is separate from the person or animal it is inhabiting is to fail to see the entire system and how the regulatory, protective process went wrong.

The condition we call cancer is a set of abnormal biological patterns driven by genetics and lifestyle; it reflects changes in the body all the way down to the microscopic and molecular levels, changes that began long before any symptoms appear or are detectable. Because a whole range of physiological processes are out of whack, it makes no sense to treat the tumor and stop there. All too often, these tumors reappear with even greater resilience and aggressiveness if the systemic condition that nurtured the original tumor is not treated. The good news is that this kind of treatment is what alternative medicine is all about.

Realizing the limitations of conventional treatment, many people have already opened their minds to other choices. A survey conducted by the American Cancer Society estimated that 9 percent of cancer patients used complementary therapies. Various other studies place the figure at 10 to 60 percent.[1] It appears that patients with cancer want integrative care, and a great majority—up to 90 percent—are using therapies other than conventional treatment.[2] Estimates by the U.S. government place annual expenditures on alternative cancer treatment for 1992 at $2 billion.[3] Americans made 425 million office visits to alternative medicine, compared to 386 million visits to conventional doctors. The Harvard study that produced these statistics also reported that at least $21.2 billion was spent on complementary and alternative medicine in 1997, at least $12.2 billion of it paid out of pocket. Furthermore, over just those few years, the volume of sales of herbal medicines and remedies increased from $30 million (1991) to $370 million (1997).[4]

That trend has only accelerated. Ten years later, according to a National Health Interview Survey conducted by the Centers for Disease Control and Prevention, adults in the United States spent $33.9 billion out of pocket on complementary and alternative medicine in 2007 alone. Approximately 83 million adults (38.3 percent) and 8.5 million children (11.8 percent) used complementary and alternative medicine in 2007.

Naturally, those who turn to alternative medicine for their own health have started looking at similar options for their pets. The most recent numbers indicate that one-fourth of pet owners have tried alternative medical treatments for their animal companions, discovering that their pets can be helped through these means effectively, safely, and inexpensively. In the case of cancer, this book will help you do all that, and it will guide you in creating an individualized program tailor-made for your pet's needs and situation. (You will find additional details, directions, and recipes in this book's appendices.)

You are your pet's only advocate. With the right information, you can help him more than you ever thought you could.

❶

TAKE CONTROL

"Your pet has cancer."

Yesterday, your dog was enthusiastically chasing a stick, your cat was happily curled up in a patch of sunshine, or your bird was sweetly trilling a song. Now, suddenly, he is a patient with that most dreaded of diseases. Panic, fear, and grief threaten to take over your life. But they don't have to. You can choose a different path to face one of the greatest challenges in your pet's life. This is what Barbara did.

In October 1997, Barbara received the biopsy report on her cat, Geronimo. Geronimo, a large, orange and white male with a placid, gentle personality, had developed a lump on the bridge of his nose. Barbara had taken him to a major teaching hospital, where the biopsy was performed. While the cat was under sedation, a surgeon removed a firm, circumscribed mass from Geronimo's face. The pathology report described a malignancy—mesenchymal neoplasia—with a "guarded" prognosis. After the surgery, the swelling between Geronimo's eyes didn't go down; in fact, the area became even more swollen, and the pus and resulting encrusted nostrils were making it difficult for the cat to breathe and, consequently, to eat.

Barbara's next step was to consult with a radiation oncologist. But two things happened on the day she took Geronimo to the hospital for his appointment. First, the appointment itself proved to be a painful eye-opener. The oncologist explained that he strongly recommended radiation treatment, not as a way to cure the cancer but merely as a way to control it. The plan he described would involve treatments five times a week for three to four weeks. The cat was likely to lose his fur, his appetite, a significant amount of weight, and perhaps his eyesight. He would develop severe skin problems in the area. Furthermore, each session would involve general anesthesia and all the risks associated with that. If Barbara decided against the treatment, the oncologist said the cat's prognosis was poor, but he could give no guarantee that radiation would lead to a successful outcome either. And even if the treatment was successful, Geronimo's life expectancy would be only six months. The final blow was the estimated cost of $3,000.

The second thing that happened to Barbara and her cat that day came in the form of a chance encounter with another cat owner in the hospital waiting room. The woman, on being told of Geronimo's condition, gave Barbara my name and telephone number and encouraged her to use the information.

"In tears," she wrote later in a note to the oncologist veterinarian, "I hauled a very large cat carrier through Copley Plaza shopping area since I could only find parking in their lot. It was close to Christmas, and I had to dodge throngs of people to get to Marie across the street. There, she treated Geronimo with acupuncture, herbs, and a homeopathic remedy. Within two weeks, all his swelling had gone."

It was in December that Geronimo became my patient. I gave him a series of six acupuncture treatments and put him on a regimen of herbal medicine given twice a day and a homeopathic remedy to be given once a day. It was three months before his nose area was back to normal, clear of all mucous discharge and swelling. In that period, the cat's appetite had returned, and he had gained weight.

A little more than a year later, the oncologist contacted Barbara to find out how the cat was faring. Since Barbara had documented Geronimo's treatment and progress, as well as the outcome, she was able to write back in great detail. His response read, "Thank you for the follow-up on your cat. . . . I can't tell you how pleased I am to hear that you have found such effective treatment at such a reasonable cost!" In May 1999 after her latest report, she received another note from the same doctor. "Thank you for the updated photo. I am glad to hear that Geronimo continues to thrive."

Geronimo lived for several more years. He continued to have his herbal medicine daily and his acupuncture therapy three or four times a year.

In the treatment of cancer, there are no "right" or "wrong" choices. There are many choices. Some may be better for your dog or cat than others. To be successful, all therapy must work on several levels at once: the body must be strengthened; the immune system enhanced; the organs, blood, and lymph detoxified; and cancer cells killed. Conventional therapies address the last level only; alternative therapies address all four.

Once you receive the diagnosis, you can start examining your choices. Don't feel pressured into making a decision immediately; you do have some time that can be used to seek a second opinion and to consult with an alternative practitioner. You can read this book.

With a health problem as complex as cancer, the more tools you have available, the better the prognosis. Conventional treatments, such as surgery, chemotherapy, and radiation, may be able to eliminate the problem, but even in a remission, some residual, undetectable cancer cells likely remain. Therefore, it's not only important but also an absolute necessity for any patient—animal or human—to begin treatment as prepared as possible. And it is just as vital to be as aggressive as possible about controlling problems that can arise during treatment and to continue working throughout and after treatment to reduce the chance of further cancerous growth and spread.

Just imagine fighting a war for 39 years with limited victories and no end in sight. This picture describes the "war" on cancer. When President Richard Nixon declared war on the disease in 1971, he invested 69 billion federal dollars in cancer research. To this date, researchers still don't know enough about cancer, whether it be its initiation, growth, or spread. Although deaths from cancer have declined slightly, cancer specialists say that this most likely reflects earlier detection of the cancer as well as lifestyle changes. The truth is that for many types of cancer, once the disease has spread, the patient's long-term survival is not much better than it was decades ago.

This disease consistently surprises researchers, doctors, and patients with its resiliency and complexity. New information means that a theory held for years gets debunked, and we start all over again. Take the idea of cancer cells and their necessary blood supply. Originally, it was thought that one protein was key to starting the process (called angiogenesis), but new research indicates that there may be at least six proteins helping tumors form blood vessels.

Cancer turns out to be more complicated than anyone thought. The typical pancreatic tumor has 63 genetic mutations; the average brain tumor, 60. How does any one treatment fit all these cases? Actually, it doesn't. The reality is that all tumors are very hard to treat, and it is never a certainty that the patient is free of cancer. "My belief is that if you intend to cure cancer, you must do more than just destroy the tumor. . . . The genesis of a tumor is just part of a larger process."[1]

It makes some sense to approach treatment from more than one direction, in other words, to develop an individualized program of choices.

WHY CONSIDER ALTERNATIVE THERAPIES?

A significant minority of cancer patients and companions to animals with cancer seek out alternatives to conventional care. The American Cancer Society gives a conservative estimate that 9 percent of U.S. cancer patients use complementary therapies, but researchers place a higher figure of up to 60 percent.[2]

The trend is worldwide. According to a survey conducted at the Women's and Children's Hospital in South Australia, approximately 36 percent of children with cancer had used at least one complementary therapy in addition to conventional treatment. In a German study of 160 cancer outpatients, 53 percent had used complementary therapies. In a survey of 949 oncology cancer outpatients from several hospitals in Holland, 9 percent were currently using complementary therapy.[3]

This raises a number of questions, the most important one being, are these patients receiving any clinical benefits? The answer is that certain therapies, when given along with conventional therapies, have doubled survival rates. You read that right: doubled. Some of the results are extraordinary. According to one study, after surgical treatment of solid tumors, survival rates were 35 percent with no supplementation (supplementation in these cases meaning acupuncture, herbal medicine, phytonutrients, diet changes, and so on), while with supplementation the rate was 62 percent. When the treatment plan included chemotherapy as well, the survival rate was 27 percent without supplementation and 53 percent with supplementation. Results such as these might make you wonder why such therapies are not more frequently mentioned or suggested by doctors.[4]

There are two approaches to combination therapy: one uses several holistic modalities in combination with conventional therapy, while the second calls for the use of holistic treatment alone. Both choices will be explored in this book. If the tumor is well defined and has all the characteristics of a tumor that can be removed successfully with surgery, without concern for metastasis, surgery appears to be a good strategy. If the tumor's margins (edges) are not clear, the outcome is murkier. Chemotherapy and/ or radiation would be advised, and these tactics run the risk of being less successful while giving rise to additional problems.

The goal of cancer treatment is to eliminate as much of the disease as possible. Surgery may remove all visible cancer, but some microscopic cancer cells can remain. Subsequent treatment is often advised. The purpose of chemotherapy and radiation is to keep the disease from returning by ridding the body of the invisible cancer cells. Both therapies are harsh and toxic; they need to be to do the job. However, pairing natural agents and treatment strategies with them will reduce their toxicity and minimize such side effects as nausea and vomiting; bowel changes; fatigue; nerve, kidney, and heart damage; urinary tract infections; mouth sores; and loss of appetite. Many types of alternative medicines, when paired with conventional treatments, make these therapies tolerable and reduce their risk, thereby leading to a significantly better outcome for patients. Determining what goes with which, that is, how cytoprotectants (the alternative medicine elements of these pairings) are matched to conventional therapies, is based on ongoing clinical research.

Chemotherapy drugs target fast-dividing cells, but these drugs can't tell a healthy fast-dividing cell from an abnormal fast-dividing one, so all are killed. Among the normal fast-dividing cells are those in the gastrointestinal tract. When they are destroyed by chemotherapy, the results are nausea, lesions in the stomach and intestines, yeast overload, and other very unpleasant and often dangerous effects. Another normal type of fast-growing cell can be found in the bone marrow. The result of killing these is a dangerous drop in red and white blood cell counts. If the toxic effects are bad enough, the oncologist may be forced to stop treatment. This can give the tumor time to regroup and begin growing back. Cytoprotectants spare the patient from these toxic side effects; they have saved many a full chemotherapy regimen from being stopped.

Even though mainstream medicine has not embraced the idea of pairing natural compounds, diet, acupuncture, herbal medicine, phytonutrients, and so on with drugs, studies and research work as well as clinical results suggest that such pairing is effective. Matching specific natural agents with specific drugs has a rationale and a purpose. There are couplings that mitigate the toxicity of particular chemotherapy drugs. Anyone justifiably terrified of chemotherapy and reluctant to give permission for its use on her animal may change her mind once she is informed of this option.

Pairings enhance the effectiveness of conventional cancer drugs; coupling makes cancer cells more susceptible to these drugs. This is important because cancer cells can acquire resistance to chemotherapy drugs; many solid tumors show a good initial response but return later in a more resistant form. A tiny number of resistant cells then have a clear path to even greater proliferation. Some pairing agents focus on supporting the action of specific cancer drugs, while others are used to increase the overall effectiveness of conventional treatment. All lead to a better outcome and help explain why patients integrating the conventional with the alternative and natural have a better prognosis.

The United States ranks among the top three countries with the highest cancer rate in humans. We have almost no statistics for companion animals. One of the foremost causes of this increase is the everyday toxic overload we—humans and animals—are exposed to. A joint study by Mount Sinai School of Medicine, Commonweal, and the Environmental Working Group in 2003 identified a total of 167 hazardous compounds. Of these, 76 are known to cause cancer, 94 are toxic to the nervous system, 82 damage the lungs, 86 affect hormone functions, and 79 cause birth defects. In each of us and in our pets, no matter where we live—be it urban or rural—the average total load is 91. No one escapes. The insult even begins in utero, according to a 2004 study that found a total of 287 industrial chemicals in babies' umbilical cord blood, 181 of these known to cause cancer. In almost every autopsy performed, cancer, although not necessarily the cause of death, is discovered.

Over the course of our lives, cancer cells develop continually; the average normal cell takes from 100 to 10,000 DNA "hits," or breaks in sequencing, every day. All these hits are potentially cancer causing. Thanks to our immune systems, most of these will not end up as cancer; our innate immunity will recognize and destroy these abnormalities before any damage is done. However, if the damaged cell is not dealt with, it ends up with two defining properties: the cell's growth pattern is completely changed and can no longer divide and differentiate normally, and its development is so altered that it acquires the ability to grow its own blood supply, invade surrounding tissues (killing off its neighbors), and travel to distant organs to seed new cancer sites.

A PLAN OF ACTION

When your pet is diagnosed with cancer, you need to develop a plan of action. Conventional cancer care may be a good and necessary option, but that alone is not sufficient. If surgery is your choice, it needs to be supported with the appropriate alternative therapeutic backup. If you decide to go with a conventional program of chemotherapy and/or radiation, pairing these steps with alternative therapies is another option. If you opt against conventional care, your program will involve choosing and employing alternative therapies. Whatever you choose, the last part of your plan should focus on helping to ensure remission from the cancer over the long term. With a plan in place, you have the power to influence your pet's outcome.

Realize that you can take charge. When a difficult choice has to be made, no one but you can assume its burden. You need to find doctors and practitioners who recognize that you have the right to disagree as well as to agree with them. Take advantage of available networks of informed people who have gone through similar difficulties. This can be a quick way to get information about which practitioners and which therapies have helped others and their pets. Of course, it is always possible that you will end up with too many people recommending too many different approaches. So here are some helpful suggestions:

- Don't assume that mainstream cancer care is the only way to go. These therapies are the same as those used on humans, and they are used aggressively. From an international perspective, American cancer therapy is considered to be extremely aggressive compared to approaches used in other countries, yet the success rate is not that much greater.
- Don't assume that all conventional treatment is effective. Statistics have consistently shown that 50 percent of individuals diagnosed with cancer survive for five years. The best success rate is associated with surgery, which depends on early detection and, when possible, cutting the entire cancer out. There remains debate in the conventional

medical community about just how much chemotherapy and radiation have contributed to human survival rates.

- Be aware of variations in competence and commitment among individual practitioners. It's common for an individual to put less effort into choosing an appropriate practitioner and therapy for himself or his pet than into choosing a new car. That's not as surprising as it sounds; most of us feel unqualified or incompetent when it comes to making medical decisions.
- Talk to pet owners about their experiences. Do go by reputation; someone who is good consistently will be good for you as well. Dare to ask your veterinarian; there is usually talk among them about who is doing what in the field. Once you've identified someone you think you could work with, be sure to ask how much formal education and experience the practitioner has had in the modality she is practicing. As a rule, someone who has studied traditional Chinese medicine, which encompasses herbal medicine and acupuncture, has had three or more years of graduate class and clinic work and has taken a comprehensive two-day national examination to be licensed in the field. A duly qualified naturopath has had four or more years of graduate study in nutrition, supplements, herbal medicines, and more. A homeopath would also have had three or more years of formal study to be seriously able to work a case. If your pet is to benefit from a nonconventional medical approach, you need to work with a knowledgeable practitioner who can make an intelligent examination and evaluation of the animal's needs and who has the experience to see a case through from beginning to end.
- Once you have made a decision, don't stop there. Continue to evaluate how the relationship between you and the medical provider and between your pet and the medical provider is going. You want someone sincerely concerned about both your pet's health needs and your emotional, economic, and philosophic needs. It is common for a veterinarian in general practice to refer a pet with cancer to a major teaching hospital or to someone specializing in oncology. If this happens, ask a lot of questions before proceeding with treatment. Avoid getting yourself into a situation in which you're dealing with hospital staff who are more concerned with the "case" than with your individual animal.

- Take a week or two to settle on a decision. It's only in very rare cases that this short time will jeopardize a pet treatment plan or the outcome. A cancer diagnosis leaves any pet owner feeling frightened, upset, and overwhelmed—not the best state of mind for making major decisions. Instead of rushing, take the time to gather information and begin to formulate a general idea of what you want to happen.

Unfortunately, the most neglected phase of cancer treatment involves preparedness. Your pet has a chronic condition; it has been in development for some time and has already used up much of his resources. He may have low, even severely depleted, white and red blood cells. He may lack vitality. He may have lost his appetite and some weight. He may even be depressed. How will being in such a state affect his chances of coming through surgery successfully? How will it affect his ability to obtain optimum results from a chemotherapy regimen?

You can prepare yourself and your pet with a self-care program put together from the information in this book as well as from other sources. You *can* start a medical partnership. You *can* begin using alternative therapies. You *can* make a difference in your pet's well-being.

Learn what you can do. Then do it all. Do it intensely. Do it repeatedly. Do it now.

2

KNOW YOUR ENEMY

When the results of a biopsy bring a diagnosis of cancer, a profound change takes place. That label—"cancer patient"—explodes like a grenade, upending everything that was once normal and casting shards of negative effects throughout your and your animal's life.

Whereas once your pet was "healthy," now he is "sick." But maybe that's not the best way to look at it. If you agree that what we call "health" exists on a continuum, then your pet is neither completely healthy nor entirely ill. He can have fine days and even very fine days, and he can have days when he is dragging around and listless. A diagnosis *is* useful, however, as a label that tells us in a very broad way what to look for, what to expect, and whether something is typically curable or incurable. Bear in mind, however, that, as a label, it is a singular lens trying to capture multiple phenomena—some pertinent to the disease, some not. A diagnosis describes averages: average experiences or average outcomes. In light of each creature's variability, it cannot sum up the identity, condition, and potential of any individual patient. A cancer label should, instead, be used as a starting point to ask additional questions and seek alternative answers.

You may be someone who rarely thinks to question a doctor's orders. But remember that you know your cat or dog better than his medical practitioner will ever be able to. You know your pet's unique history as well as his physical and emotional makeup, so you can, with enough information and thought, know which treatment options are most likely to suit him. Your satisfaction with the treatment he gets will depend on how it serves his unique needs and not that of some statistically generalized patient. Knowing the most vital aspects of your pet as you do, you need to listen most carefully to yourself. Medical professionals are the experts on the general course of an illness and treatment, but we are the experts on our and our pet's individual journey.

Now, if you're going to lead this fight against cancer on behalf of your pet, you need to know your enemy. Cancer is not one single disease. Cancer takes hundreds of different forms, all bearing the same fundamental characteristic: damage to cellular DNA. Once this damage begins, a cancerous cell ends up with two defining properties: the cell is completely changed and can no longer divide and differentiate normally, and its development is so altered that it has acquired the ability to invade surrounding tissues and travel to distant sites.

A damaged cell undergoes a process involving three steps: initiation, promotion, and progression. The initiation period begins when a cell becomes exposed to some triggering substance or event during its replication process. Some exposures are environmental in nature, such as a virus, a toxic chemical, or radiation—all capable of setting the cell off on its malignant journey. Initiation can also be started by a long-term, chronic problem, such as inflammation; many cancers have an underlying inflammatory component.

At initiation, the body's own enzyme defenses will usually detect errors in DNA replication and block further cell division. The error will either be repaired or the cell will be told to self-destruct. But if the error is missed, it becomes a permanent mutation. And because it looks "normal," the cancerous cell is left to its own devices.

The second step in the cancer process is exposure to factors that promote its growth. Promoters include toxins, such as additives and chemicals in food and drinking water; prescription drugs; hormones; indoor and outdoor air pollution; lifestyle factors; certain occupational hazards; and, of course, a suppressed immune system or the absence of innate immune activity that results from chronic disease, aging, extreme stress, or certain long-term infections. Theoretically, cancer can start and progress when any one (or more) of these factors arrives on the scene.

Cancer researchers find the first stage of initiation particularly intriguing, as if they could develop a nearly foolproof surveillance system or provide the body with the tools it needs to disrupt the DNA changes, most cancer initiation could be stopped in its tracks. But to counter the initiation process, such a surveillance system would need to have two major elements in optimum working order: the cell-mediated immune response and the humoral immune response.

The cell-mediated immune response protects the body against bacterial, viral, and fungal infections primarily through the actions of the T-lymphocytes. The humoral immune response involves antibodies acquired through earlier life encounters with foreign pathogens or through vaccinations and responds through the activity of the B-lymphocytes. Together, these two parts of the immune system serve the body by providing antibody production, cellular immunity, and immunological memory.

Cancer cells carry markings called surface antigens; these are specialized protein molecules that trigger an immune response. When the T-lymphocytes of the immune system encounter these antigens (tumor-associated antigens and tumor-specific antigens), they start releasing chemicals called lymphokines that begin to destroy the cell surface. During this process, these lymphokines are themselves transformed into the "killer" T-lymphocytes. These cells then finish the destruction process. This route is called the cell-mediated immune response.

A humoral immune response also depends on recognition of a cancer cell's surface antigens, in this case, tumor-specific antigens. An antigen binds with the B-lymphocyte antigen receptor and initiates a response. Once the antigen is recognized, antibodies are released into the plasma cells, and, this time, it is the B-lymphocytes that will do the destroying. The activated antibodies, now differentiated into plasma cells and under the direction of the B-lymphocytes, create immunoglobulins, notably the interleukins and interferons often talked about in cancer treatment.

No system is fail-safe, however. If the immune system fails to recognize a tumor cell as abnormal or "foreign," the immune response won't activate. The tumor will continue to grow until it is beyond the system's ability to destroy it. The inability to recognize, react to, and eliminate abnormalities is often due to a disruption in or a suppression of the immune system. Indeed, the tumor cell itself can suppress immune defenses by changing the appearance of its antigens, thus successfully hiding itself.

The rapid, uncontrollable proliferation of cells and the ability to spread from its area of origin to a secondary site anywhere in the body are the two fundamental characteristics of cancer. The dispersal of cells occurs through ordinary circulation via the bloodstream and/or through lymphatic tissue fluid. Growth can also occur through the extension of the abnormal cells into surrounding tissue.

A major part of the body's protection lies in a cell's internal clock. Every healthy cell has a mechanism that tells it when it's time to reproduce, lie dormant, or die. Cancer cells have no such control. Unrestrained, they go through cell growth stages much faster than normal. Every aspect of cell activity changes as a result: cell shape, organization, structure, membrane, adhesion, and permeability. Chaos rules. Communication between cells becomes impaired, and recognition of other cells is diminished. In order to perpetuate this uncontrolled proliferation, cancer cells need a vast supply of nutrients.

In a normal cell, internal cell control occurs through the activity of specific regulator genes or proteins that act as on-and-off switches. Different cells respond to special control genes; for example, there is a control gene called "c-myc" that helps to begin DNA replication. If this gene senses an error in DNA replication, it tells the cell to self-destruct.

Other factors, such as hormones, also affect gene control activity. (The hormone erythropoietin is one; it stimulates red blood cell production.) In cancer cells, however, control devices are either lacking or defective.

Communication between cells that are close to each other is necessary for them to share information about neighboring cells and the amount of space available for future growth. If an area is crowded, the nearest cells will signal other cells to slow down or even cease reproduction. Cancer cells fail to recognize these signals, instead crowding out their neighbors with their uncontrolled growth, cutting off their neighbors' blood supply, and killing them.

Unlike normal cells, cancer cells can develop finger-like projections that help in this destructive process; these projections attach to the walls of normal cells, breaking through their membranes and taking over. The abnormal cell thus completes its initiation period, progressing to a larger mass and moving part of itself into a new home.

All normal cells differentiate, becoming specialized and developing very individualized characteristics that prepare them for their roles in the body. As cells become more and more specialized, their reproduction and development slows down; eventually, highly differentiated cells become unable to reproduce and are programmed to die and be replaced. Skin cells are one example.

Cancer cells do not differentiate. Instead, they enter a state called anaplasia, losing the appearance and function of the original cell. The permeability of cancer cells' membranes is altered to allow much greater amounts of nutrients to flow in and feed the demands of rapid growth. The nuclei become huge and odd shaped. Breaks, deletions, and chromosomal defects are typical.

CANCER TYPES AND TIMING

Ordinarily, a long time passes between the initiation period and the onset of the disease. How fast the tumor grows depends on its specific characteristics and on the host. Among the characteristics are location and available blood supply. Where the tumor cell happens to be will also influence its growth. If it's a fast-growing site, such as in the epithelial layers, cancer grows rapidly. If it's in connective tissue, it grows more slowly. Cancer cells need their own blood supply to provide the nutrients and oxygen for their growth and the removal of wastes. Some solve the problem by growing their own blood vessels, a process called angiogenesis. Some produce their own growth factors. Either way, the tumor grows.

As for the host, it appears that age is the single most common, important factor affecting tumor growth. The incidence of cancer correlates directly with increasing age. Of course, it's likely that there are numerous and accumulative events that may be necessary for the initial mutation to arise, continue, and eventually form a tumor. That is why the overall health of the host is vital—because it can alter normal body processes. A factor such as a nutritional deficiency can create an environment in which opportunities for initiation multiply.

When cancer cells survive long enough to reach 1 to 2 millimeters in mass, they require additional blood vessels for continued growth and mutation. At that size, the tumor mass extends into local tissues, and, if the local tissues are blood or lymph, the tumor can gain access to a circulation system perfect for metastasis. By breaking off parts of itself, the tumor sends cancerous cells to other sites in the body—via ordinary circulation in the bloodstream and through lymphatic tissue fluid—where they will settle in to grow and form additional tumors. Cancer that doubles in 60 days is considered the most aggressive, cancer that doubles in 61 to 150 days is labeled moderately aggressive, and cancer that doubles in 151 to

300 days is called indolent. Extremely indolent cancer has a doubling time of more than 300 days.

Just to give you some perspective on the problem, the average size of a human breast cancer when first detected by mammography is about 600 million cells, about one-quarter inch across. A similar tumor found by manual palpation has about 45 billion cells and appears to be one and a quarter inches in size.

Invasive tumor cells usually lodge in a readily available capillary bed. The lungs are a perfect place and are a very common site for metastasis. In the new site, the tumor cells develop a protective coating to evade detection by the immune system. Once settled in, the tumor begins to invade its new neighbors. If the tumor cells enter the lymph system, they can be transported to distant sites, then trapped in the fluid. Subsequent enlargement of a lymph node can be evidence of metastasis or a localized reaction to the tumor. Whether through the bloodstream or the multitude of connections between the two systems—blood and lymph—the tumor has spawned its offspring.

Malignant tumors are classified by the type of tissue in which the growth originated, that is, the three cell layers that form our bodies during the early stages of embryonic development: the ectoderm, the mesoderm, and the endoderm. The ectoderm forms the external embryonic coverings and structures that will come into contact with the environment, such as the skin. The endoderm becomes the inner lining of many systems, and the mesoderm forms the circulatory, urinary, reproductive, and muscular structures, plus their supporting tissues. A carcinoma is a tumor of either endodermal or ectodermal origin and is labeled an adenocarcinoma. A sarcoma originates in the mesoderm.

Malignant tumors are also graded and classified by their degree of differentiation. This ranges from grade 1, in which the cells still closely resemble the tissue of origin, through to less and less differentiation, and, ultimately, to grade 4, which has no resemblance to the tissue of origin. Malignant tumors are further classified anatomically. This is called staging, a process that evaluates tumor size, nodal involvement, and metastatic progress. Staging provides a useful description of the tumor, pointing the way toward appropriate treatment and prognosis.

Any treatment must try to disrupt the initiation, promotion, and/or progression of the cancer. Any cancer therapy has one or more of the following goals: to eradicate the cancer and promote long-term survival, to control or arrest the growth of the cancerous cells, to alleviate symptoms (palliation) when the disease is beyond control, and prophylaxis for high-risk tumor development. All the conventional treatments may be used alone or in combination (an approach called multimodal), depending on the tumor's size, state, site, predicted responsiveness to treatment, and, of course, any limitations stemming from the patient's clinical state.

Alternative medicine regards cancer as a manifestation of a body whose defensive systems are so severely impaired that they cannot destroy cells that have turned abnormal, that is, as a systemic, not a localized, disease. Because it's a whole-body disease, a comprehensive program is required, one that utilizes as many tools as possible to help fight the cancer. The best chance for a remission lies in the use of alternative therapies, whatever conventional treatments are employed. Among the most important of these is traditional Chinese medicine, which includes acupuncture and herbal medicine. Add to this a truly good nutrition program, along with Western herbal medicine, supplements, and homeopathy, and you have a complete plan.

Currently, one out of three humans will be diagnosed with cancer at some point in their lives. In most cases, they will be treated by the same methods that have been used for decades. The statistics for pets are lacking, but from the looks of things, they are not too far behind us. The World Health Organization has long predicted that cancer would overtake heart disease as the developed world's leading cause of death. It is up to you to change the odds—for you and your pet.

There are five major types of cancer:

- *Carcinomas* are usually found in the epithelial cells that cover the surface of the skin, mouth, nose, throat, lung airways, and genital, urinary, and gastrointestinal tracts or that line glands such as the breast and thyroid. Lung, breast, prostate, skin, stomach, and colon cancers are called carcinomas and are solid tumors.
- *Sarcomas* are those that form in the bones and in the soft connective and supportive tissues surrounding organs and tissues, such as cartilage, muscle, tendons, fat, and the outer linings of the lungs, abdomen, heart, nervous system, and blood vessels. Sarcomas are solid tumors and are the rarest and most deadly.
- *Leukemias* form in the blood and bone marrow; the abnormal white blood cells travel through the bloodstream, often causing problems in

the spleen. They are not solid tumors but rather an overproduction of abnormal white blood cells.

- *Lymphomas* are cancers of the lymph glands. The lymph glands act as a filter for the body's impurities and are concentrated in the neck, groin, armpits, spleen, the center of the chest, and around the intestines. Lymphomas are made up of abnormal lymphocytes, which are white blood cells that congregate in the lymph glands and form solid tumors.
- *Myelomas* are rare and come from antibody-producing plasma cells—the red cells—in the bone marrow.

For precursors to cancer, see Appendix A.

3

THE TERRAIN IS EVERYTHING

Researching into plants and other natural materials for anticancer activity and subsequent use in therapy began in 1955 with funding from the National Cancer Institute. The original mission was to develop new agents for treatment, and, although the project started off slowly, by 1991 more than 114,000 plant samples representing 4,000 species internationally had been screened. In reality, this represents a mere 2 percent of the world's approximately 250,000 plant species. Research centers sponsored by other governments have also been actively searching for botanical anticancer agents.[1]

Successful searches for anticancer agents face monumental problems. First, cancer is not one single disease but can present as nearly 200 distinct types, with each type behaving quite differently. Ideally, research would have to include multiple cancers, but this proves expensive and time consuming. In addition, for many years, such research was not even technologically feasible.

Until recently, cancer cells have been identified primarily as fast growing; as such, they have been treated in a variety of ways, including surgery, radiation, and chemotherapy. Chemotherapy agents now in use are toxic to both cancerous and normal fast-growing cells (such as the gastrointestinal lining and bone marrow cells). The focus on destroying fast-growing cells has resulted in a lack of research into other agents that might be active against the most common cancers, which are, in many cases, slower growing.

The ability to identify new agents that may work well against proliferating cancer cells is also complicated by the fact that these agents appear to work through multiple mechanisms. So even if it is identified as active, the mechanism by which it works may remain unknown.

In the meantime, many cancer cell lines and individual cancers have mutant subpopulations that are resistant to any form of treatment and are able to continue to proliferate. This characteristic can render them difficult to breed for experimental testing purposes, while otherwise effective anticancer agents are useless against them.

Large amounts of plant material are needed to meet the needs of clinical trials, to determine their usefulness as anticancer agents, making the screening process difficult and expensive. As a result, in vitro screening (in an artificial environment, such as in a test tube) is used much more frequently, although it is not as effective as in vivo screening (within a living organism) in identifying agents on one primary action, their cytotoxicity, or the ability to kill cancer cells.

In 1991, the National Cancer Institute began a multidisciplinary approach in testing plant and marine organism materials from around the world that could yield new cancer chemoprevention activity.[2] A fraction of these have received marketing approval by the U.S. Food and Drug Administration. However, no botanical should be written off. Not all plant-derived anticancer agents are discovered by the National Cancer Institute's screening process. The anticancer properties of vinblastine and vincristine, both used extensively in cancer treatment, were derived from the periwinkle plant grown in Madagascar and discovered by accident during research on antidiabetic activity. The popular drug Adriamycin as well as actinomycin D and mitomycin D, teniposide, and etoposide were products of non–cancer-related research and derived from botanical agents.[3]

While the complete story of how natural agents work against cancer is not currently known, we do have some answers. Some botanicals work to stimulate DNA repair mechanisms, preventing further abnormal development. Others produce antioxidant effects by scavenging after free radicals. Some promote the production of protective chemicals, such as the enzymes glutathione peroxidase, reductase, and transferase. Some inhibit cancer-activating enzymes and circulating immune complexes. Some cause cancer cell death through increasing oxygen. Whatever their roles in cancer treatment, phytochemicals can be powerful tools if applied and used appropriately.

Although many of the alternative methods for treating cancer have been with us for some 40 years, it is only in the past two decades that these approaches have moved into wider public awareness. A great deal of what you read here will probably be new to you and your veterinarian. He may not know more than the very basics of nutrition, the immune system, and herbal medicine. Conventional veterinary medical schools (and medical schools in general) hardly ever discuss these topics; as a consequence, the practitioner may remain in the conventional box, not looking beyond to see what might work better. Even when information about alternative approaches to cancer reaches him, he often seems to pay it little attention. Most conventional veterinarians ignore the results when accepted treatments such as chemotherapy fail and refuse to change their methods. They also frequently ignore the successful results that occur when their patients have switched to nonconventional care.

Many factors contribute to the development of cancer, and just as many modalities and substances are needed to reverse it. Alternative medical practitioners believe that to be successful in eliminating cancer, they must become generalists and address the whole body, treating nutritional and dietary needs as well as the vitality of the patient and his immune system. And they believe that they must be willing to adjust their therapies accordingly. There is a famous saying: science and medicine advance funeral by funeral. Old beliefs and practices eventually die out, giving way to new approaches. The time has come for the greater use of complementary/alternative medical treatments for cancer.

Primary Complements and Alternatives to Chemotherapy

Metabolic enzymes
Glandulars
Metabolic antioxidants
Probiotics
Metabolic amino acids
Homeopathic remedies
Metabolic herbals and botanicals
Essential fatty acids
Vitamins and minerals
Sea vegetables
Fiber supplements

Primary Programs

Nutritional support
Immune system modification
Constitutional support
Liver, bowel, blood, and/or lymph detoxification

4

BEGIN WITH FOOD

Much of what can be done for cancer requires a level of medical and technological skill and expertise that is beyond the realm of the average person's experience. What you can do, however, is put in place a strong supporting program of alternative options, a nutritional supplement program, and the inclusion of micronutrients, such as vitamins, minerals, enzymes, amino acids, and so on. Using several or all of these unconventional therapies lets you address a number of immediate and long-term problems affecting your pet. These may include rebuilding a weakened immune system or healing injured organs, such as the liver, kidneys, and gastrointestinal tract. The more complicated therapies need the guidance of professionals; working with an acupuncturist, herbalist, and homeopath will help your pet get through surgery, conventional chemotherapy, and/or radiation therapy with a minimum of problems and enhance the effects of conventional treatment significantly.

The case of Robert, a large, handsome Doberman of seven years, can help shed light on how such a program can work. Robert had been raised, like most dogs, on a conventional processed diet. His owner found a suspicious lump in Robert's right rear leg that turned out to be an osteosarcoma. The dog underwent a series of X-rays to determine if any of the tumor had metastasized. Because there was no sign of cancer anywhere, the decision was made to amputate the leg.

Robert adjusted well postsurgically and finished all the conventional drugs, but his owner was concerned about the future. What she wanted was some insurance that the cancer would stay in remission and that Robert would live out his remaining years disease free, pain free, and happy. When Robert and I met, all his vital signs and blood work appeared normal. I suggested to his owner that our work together could be to first develop a great food plan and then to supplement it with herbs, other nutrients, and acupuncture. Since the owner was excited about the role of food in cancer prevention, she agreed to feed Robert home-cooked food every day. Her choice of menu alternated between organically raised chicken and wild salmon, either baked or grilled, with vegetables chosen in season and from a wide variety of colors and tastes, finished off with a small amount of grain. Both chicken and salmon would provide good protein without huge amounts of calories since now that Robert was a large but only a three-legged dog, he had to remain lean. To keep inflammation down, she added several types of fruits and vegetables known for their anti-inflammatory and antioxidant properties. I recommended Chinese herbal medicine: one formula to address the possibility of abnormal cells developing and another to keep his immune system at optimum levels. Finally, we arranged an ongoing schedule of acupuncture every 8 to 10 weeks. This last would keep Robert healthy in many different ways: it would boost his energy and his immune system and keep strain on the remaining three legs and joints minimal. With all this in place, Robert lived several more years cancer free. Robert's case is an example of a comprehensive program that utilizes as many tools as necessary. Robert needed only the surgery to rid his body of cancer, but for others with either different kinds of cancer or the possibility that the disease is present in more than one site, additional conventional therapies would be employed. In these cases, combining conventional treatments with complementary therapies in an integrative system buys the best odds for a successful outcome.

The pet in this situation has nutritional needs that include cancer-fighting nutrients such as phytochemicals (plant chemicals), in addition to good protein, essential fats, and healthy fluids. If your pet goes into treatment with weight and muscle loss, decreased appetite, and what would be considered cachexia (wasting syndrome), he will need a nutrition plan that will stop this downward spiral. Cachexia results from high levels of inflammatory biochemicals, which are secreted by cancer cells. Cachexia ceases when a tumor shrinks or is killed off.

Unintentional, uncontrolled weight loss can mean that muscles waste away and the immune system weakens, raising the risk of life-threatening infections. The more malnourished the patient, the more suppressed the immune system, also resulting in a heightened susceptibility to metastasis. Human cancer patients have a very high prevalence of malnutrition second only to AIDS patients; nearly half of all patients suffering from advanced-stage cancers suffer from malnutrition-related complications. It's no different with our pets. However, loading up the patient with calories is not an option. Instead, you must optimize the nutritional state of your pet, and this in turn will influence cell stability and return tumor-promoting molecules to a more normal state, keeping proliferation under control. You can even incite cancer cell death, called apoptosis, through food and supplements. This chapter and those that follow empower you to help your pet through what inevitably follows from conventional cancer care.

Let's begin with food. Food is one of the critical foundations at the heart of health and energy. Because food is so important, we should pay attention to it. The rich array of hundreds of available food compounds give us ways to keep ourselves and our pets healthy or, if sick, to heal.

The practice of using food as medicine can be traced throughout history. All societies included food as part of their healing rituals. Food frequently complemented medical care, and food is still respected for its health-giving and health-maintaining value. In most cultures, the kitchen is the first line of defense against simple, acute illness. The congees, soups, teas, porridge, elixirs, and tonics that Mom brewed on the stove gave babies their first experiences with the medicinal effects of food. Including your pet in a wholesome food program is one of the best gifts you can give him.

It is for good reason that nutrition is one of the first considerations in a treatment plan. Because nutrients are basic to the cellular environment, the use of nutrients as therapy for healing is based on the wide role that these macronutrients and micronutrients have in cell structure and chemistry. Many, if not most, diseases have a nutritional deficiency aspect, and this is the place to start the healing. Good nutrition provides both the environment and the tools.

The best foods are the ones over which you have some control. The ingredients you use can be top quality, chosen in season, and freshly cooked with methods that ensure retention of nutrients. And you can supplement home-cooked meals with herbs, remedies, and other bioregulators to enhance the effects. When starting a pet on a home-cooked diet, remember that variety and simplicity are key. Start cautiously. Begin with a very few ingredients simmered in a broth; as your dog or cat adapts to the new food, you can gradually add more and different ingredients.

Food needs to be fresh and whole: fresh because in-season fruits and vegetables are at their peak of nutrient availability and whole because all of us—human and animal—are designed to benefit from the synergistic components of individual foods and food combinations. Fresh fruit and vegetables contain enzymes, proteins, and hundreds of other components that are interconnected and interdependent. Artificially created substances, synthetic vitamins and minerals, processed foods, and poorly prepared food are all incomplete, stripped of or isolated from their original context. These foods often lead to negative consequences on our health.

Let's begin by talking about proteins. The most typical source of protein—red meat—has been linked to cancer by scientists: eating two servings of red meat a day is associated with four times the risk of problems. In general, what's wrong with meat is its high amount of omega-6 fatty acids, which are converted into inflammatory molecules that fuel tumor growth. Diets rich in meat boost the level of estradiol, an estrogen hormone that stimulates the growth of certain tumors. Red meats are also high in iron, causing the body to generate many more free radicals than normal, in turn causing more DNA damage. (Free radicals and their role in cancer are discussed in a later chapter.)

Proteins are essential nutrients; they provide enzymes that are the spark plugs to chemical processes. They also are necessary in the production of certain hormones, neurotransmitters, and antibodies, and they make up organs such as skin, hair, fur, nails, and muscle. Protein deficiencies can lead to a lack of development or abnormalities in development in almost all parts of the body. A good protein is easy to digest and well utilized. But, in excess, proteins are inefficiently assimilated and can increase the level of internal toxicity. The key to maintaining a balance is to select a variety of proteins from all sources: animal, fish, and plant. If you select fish, choose wild as opposed to farm-raised fish; if meat, free range, uncontaminated, and fed from organic, clean sources. As much as possible, buy from suppliers you can trust.

Several kinds of fat—saturated, polyunsaturated, and monounsaturated—are all essential to health in varying degrees. The most common problem with them lies in the amount and type of fat. If consumed in moderation, all fats, except trans-fatty acids, are health promoting and the most concentrated source of energy you can find. Fats, or lipids, constitute the main component of cell membranes and are regulators of specific metabolic processes, such as the production of neurotransmitters. Fats also aid in the absorption of fat-soluble vitamins (such as vitamins A and D) and make calcium bioavailable.

Many people are confused about the difference between a "good" fat and a "bad" one. Fat is composed of one glycerol molecule linked with three fatty acid molecules. That's why it's called a "triglyceride." A fatty acid molecule is a chain of carbon, oxygen, and hydrogen atoms. The number of hydrogen atoms can vary, but if the molecule has its full capacity of hydrogen atoms, it is "saturated." Unsaturated molecules have missing hydrogen atoms; if two are missing, it is called monounsaturated; if four or more are missing, it is called polyunsaturated. Fats from animal sources contain mostly saturated fatty acids, whereas vegetable oils are typically unsaturated. Saturated fat forces the liver to produce more low-density lipoprotein (LDL), the vehicle that carries cholesterol to and through the arteries. LDL promotes the buildup of atherosclerotic plaque, or deposits, on the artery walls and inhibits blood circulation.

Using a product labeled "pure vegetable oil" is not the answer to healthier cooking. The oil could have been made in large part from highly saturated oils. Monounsaturated and polyunsaturated oils tend to lower the amount of LDL in the body. Monounsaturated oil has an edge over the polyunsaturated type because it doesn't decrease the amount of high-density lipoprotein (HDL), the "good" cholesterol. Vegetable oils are made of both mono- and polyunsaturated fats; it's the percentage of the mix that's important. Tropical oils have the highest ratios of saturated to unsaturated fat. Popular oils such as canola, walnut, safflower, corn, sunflower, sesame, and olive oils can range from 6 percent saturated to 15 percent saturated to mono- and polyunsaturated. Olive oil and canola oil have the highest percentage of monounsaturated fat, while safflower, sunflower, and soybean have the highest polyunsaturated percentage.

Having cancer increases the body's need for micronutrients (such as vitamins and minerals). If you decide to have your pet treated conventionally, his micronutrient needs will skyrocket. Radiotherapy and chemotherapy drugs use free radicals to kill tumors; this, in turn, raises the body's demand for antioxidants. Studies have shown lower mortality and recurrence rates for patients who had high dietary antioxidants.[1] Where do these come from? Foods such as kale, spinach, strawberries, blueberries, blackberries, cranberries, and raspberries have an antioxidant capacity of over 100. Prunes, plums, red peppers, beets, Brussels sprouts, and broccoli have an antioxidant capacity of over 60.

As you can see, plants are the answer to the antioxidant question. The nutrients from plants do fantastic work for the body. They modulate tumor growth by affecting the workings of the genes that regulate cell division, they produce anti-inflammatory chemicals, they promote cancer cell death, and they help the body recover from chemotherapy toxicity. In general, it's a great idea to load up your pet's plate with foods high in antioxidant capacity.

THE SHOCKING TRUTH ABOUT OUR PETS' FOOD

If you have been feeding your pet commercially processed dog or cat food, you may be shocked at what is really in that bag or can. The shrimp, fish, and other marine foods grown on fish farms are probably eating "tankage" shipped from renderers who include dead dog and cat bodies as partial ingredients. Tankage is the material from rendering plants. As one president of a West Coast rendering plant told a reporter, "We've been building a mountain of euthanized cats and dogs in the back."[2] This material is included in the processing of pet food and is fed to the farmed fish and seafood that comes back for sale to the United States, mostly from Pacific Rim countries. China, one of the countries that uses tankage, is the leading exporter of seafood to the United States (China is also raising most of its fish products for human consumption in water contaminated with raw sewage and animal waste and then using dangerous chemicals—most of which are banned in the United States by the Food and Drug Administration [FDA]—to clean up the toxins.[3]) The vast number of hidden sources in the global food market system make attempts to track the ingredients and ensure their safety almost impossible. You would feed your pet better if the fish you bought were "wild caught."

In order to understand the problems presented by our food and that of our pets, we must look at what can legally go into foods, how these products are made, and how commercial food processing companies work. Unfortunately, we can't depend on our government agencies for much help.

The notion that these agencies keep our food free of harmful ingredients is a myth. Enforcement of the Delaney Amendment, which mandated that no cancer-causing additives be added to food, continues to be only superficial. There are many known carcinogens in what we and our pets eat and drink. All kinds of drugs contaminate our food supplies. More than 40 percent of the 50 million pounds of antibiotics produced in this country are used for animals. The determination that a food additive is safe is left largely to the manufacturer. Additives such as flavorings and colorings pose potential danger to various body systems. The use of pesticides, herbicides, and insecticides that are known to be cancer-causing agents continues.

Nearly two-thirds of the fish, almost one-half of the fruit, and more than 10 percent of the vegetables we eat are imported. Yet of the more than 20 billion pounds of produce we import yearly, only 2 to 3 percent undergoes FDA inspection.

It's quite likely that today's food is grown in soil that is almost entirely depleted of nutrients. In exchanging quality for quantity, growers are forced to use greater and greater amounts of chemical fertilizers. The result is that it now takes 80 cups of today's supermarket spinach to give us the same amount of iron one got from one cup of spinach 50 years ago. There is only half the protein in the wheat we eat now compared to the wheat our grandparents ate.[4]

Some 5,000 additives are currently used to color, preserve, and give texture to food. Additives are substances intentionally added during food production, processing, storage, and packaging. While a tiny amount of additives are beneficial, many more are harmful, even lethal. Most are added not for their nutritional value but to preserve our illusions of what food should look, feel, taste, and smell like.

Beautiful food in books and magazines or on television looks a certain way. Not surprisingly, you come to expect this perfect food in real life: unblemished fruits and vegetables, red (not gray) meat, and yellow egg yolks—all perfect in color, shape, and texture. Having given us the mental image of the ideal apple, carrot, or steak through advertising, food growers and processors have to then deliver food that actually approaches that ideal. They can achieve this only with the use of pesticides, herbicides, dyes, and preservatives. We want our food tasty, appealing, and easy to prepare, but we're not so concerned with its nutritional profile. No wonder the biggest category of food additives is flavorings and flavor enhancers.

Almost all commercially prepared food contains nonessential acidifiers, alkalizers, moisteners or drying agents, extenders, disinfectants, maturers, and bleaches. Additives are big business: in 2004, the U.S.

market for food additives was estimated to total $5.8 billion.[5] How many of these are truly safe?

The FDA relies heavily on manufacturers to ensure that additives work as intended and are safe for human consumption. (Almost no safeguards are imposed on pet foods.) Each year, these companies seek FDA approval of more than 100 new food additives. Safety standards are based on consumption by a healthy young male; no data are required about the effects on women, children, or pets.

Despite FDA assurances, some of the additives it has approved have been shown to cause serious health problems. Some red and yellow food dyes are allergens, and one blue dye has caused brain tumors in lab animals. The nitrates and nitrites that appear on many food labels present special problems. They combine with ammonia in the body to form carcinogenic compounds called nitrosamines. Sulfates and sulfites, often used in dairy products, grains, cereals, and preserved fruits, are also potentially dangerous. Aluminum sulfite, for example, can become a potent neurotoxin in the brain. Many foaming and defoaming agents are derived from aluminum, which has been implicated in changes in the brain leading to senility and Alzheimer's disease. Along with these nonessential ingredients, food can contain contaminants such as lead solder from cans, chemicals that leach from plastic containers, or mold that grows in stored grains and nuts.

Some additives and contaminants are known carcinogens, though no one can say for sure how much exposure to these chemicals is needed to cause cancer. Some epidemiologists estimate that about one-third of cancer deaths can be attributed to diet. Some scientists believe that neurotoxins in food that impair brain and nerve function are even more of a problem than carcinogens. Among the chemicals found in food that have been shown or are suspected to be neurotoxins are monosodium glutamate, red dye #3, and some residual pesticides.

How can you protect yourself and your pet? Are you safe if a product is labeled "organic"? Organic food regulations that took effect in 2002 specify that organic crops are those grown without the use of artificial chemicals. The U.S. Department of Agriculture's organic seal means the product is at least 95 percent organic. If the label says "made with organic ingredients," then between 70 and 95 percent of the ingredients must be organic. If less than 70 percent of a product is organic, labels can list organic ingredients, but the overall product can't be called organic.

Just four months after the new standards took effect, however, Congress passed legislation relaxing the standards to allow meat to be labeled "organic" even when it comes from livestock fed nonorganic feed, which is contaminated with antibiotics and hormones.

As with all things, additives that may not bother one person or pet may be harmful to another, especially those with food allergies or sensitivities, compromised immune systems, diabetes, high blood pressure, heart problems, or a genetic susceptibility to cancer. Manufacturers can add small amounts of allergens without listing them as ingredients, while others may be listed under misleading names. For example, a product that does not list "milk" as an ingredient may contain casein, sodium caseinate, or other constituents of milk.

There is no value difference in feeding canned or dry processed food to your pet. Canned foods tend to contain fewer preservatives than dry food, but the heat- and vacuum-packing process can decrease the integrity and quality of vitamins and minerals available in the food. Semimoist foods often contain high levels of sweeteners, preservatives, and colorings. Sweeteners in particular can stimulate the pancreas to work overtime and set the stage for pancreatic disease and the body's inability to digest food properly. Added salt can lead to fluid retention, heart disease, and stroke.

The pet food recall of 2007 brought to light the fact that many pet food companies get their lines of food from only one or two manufacturers. These lines can range from the cheapest to the highest-priced premium food, yet the product may basically contain the same inferior ingredients, or, if better ingredients are used, they may be contaminated through using the same equipment. Don't be fooled into thinking that a private-brand label means much in terms of quality.

Why is commercial pet food so bad? Pet food manufacturers are self-regulated. No government agency has major input into ingredients or regulations as they pertain to commercially made pet food. If your pet becomes ill after eating a pet food made in the United States, you can't go to the FDA and request the agency investigate. Before any action would be considered, you would have to supply scientific data that indicate the source of the problem: veterinary reports, blood work, urinalysis, other medical tests, and a chemical analysis of the questionable food. In the case of the 2007 pet food recall, the FDA waited for manufacturers and pet food companies to voluntarily recall their products. The recall took months and dragged on, while more and more companies and brand names were added to the list of offenders. Dogs and cats, meanwhile, were dying because consumers trusted their brand of pet food.

The pet food industry is a multi-billion-dollar business and a growing one. Two or three manufacturers produce the majority of the food for the large private-label pet food companies. Buying what you may consider a "better" food than the supermarket brands for your pet usually proves a waste of money. Don't depend on the pet food lining the walls of your veterinarian's clinic either; it is no better. Some of this food is sold as "prescription food" at high prices, but unless the veterinarian has training in pet nutrition, he is recommending not what he knows but what the pet food industry has sold him. Doctors for humans don't recommend or sell food products to their patients claiming that they will cure or manage a health problem.

To make sense of the problem, we have to learn to read labels. Only about half of the actual contents of a pet food, either canned or bagged, are listed on the label due to the minimal legal regulation of this industry. The words on the label are often obscure and sometimes even meaningless. For example, the term "meat by-products" can mean lungs filled with pneumonia and tuberculosis, livers infested with flukes or diseased with cirrhosis, or intestines with worms; even those areas of the body where the animals have been injected with drugs are included. It is a common practice for thousands of euthanized cats and dogs to be rendered and become part of an ingredient called "meat meal." (The bodies are thrown into rendering vats along with collars, ID tags, and plastic bags.) In the rendering process, there are no "clean" parts: fur and stomach contents are not excluded.

Poultry fares no better. Necks, feet, undeveloped eggs, and intestines are in poultry by-product meal. Poultry by-products include heads, feet, and viscera (sometimes with fecal matter still inside), and even poultry feathers. Fish ingredients are often fish heads, tails, fins, bones, and viscera. Fish meal is the rendered residue of heads, tails, innards, and blood. When the entire fish is used, it may be because the fish contains a high level of mercury or other toxins that make it unfit for human consumption.

Many other sources make up what is considered acceptable protein ingredients: hair from cattle, horses, pigs, and other slaughtered animals; animal blood, food waste, and any other animal and vegetable products picked up from institutions such as hospitals, restaurants, and grocery stores, including garbage; dehydrated garbage; animal and vegetable waste separated from glass or metal; dehydrated paunch products and digested food and water of slaughtered cattle; dried poultry waste, processed body waste matter that could contain straw or wood shavings; dried swine waste, fibers, bedding material, straw, and wood shavings;

and undried, processed animal waste product, with litter, wood shavings, dirt, sand, rocks, and similar material.

One agricultural practice is feeding poultry litter to cattle. In areas of the country where large cattle and poultry operations coexist, chicken waste is routinely fed to cows. Poultry litter consists primarily of manure, feathers, spilled feed, and bedding material that accumulates on the floors of the buildings that house chickens and turkeys. It can contain disease-causing bacteria, heavy metals, drugs such as antibiotics, and foreign objects. This practice is legal even though it is inhumane and creates unacceptable risks to human and animal health.

Grains make up a good portion of pet food. Corn is overused and may be listed on the label three or four times as corn, corn flour, corn bran, and corn gluten meal, constituting up to half of the product. Grains used this way are not good for cats, who need half their diet to be from protein, nor is it good for dogs because it offers empty calories and minimal nutrients. Wheat sources can be labeled wheat flour, middlings, shorts, and meal and can also include the floor sweepings of leftovers in the milling. Many grains in pet food contain high levels of herbicides, pesticides, and fungicides; grain sources that are not fit for human consumption are passed down for pet food inclusion.

Commercial pet food contains ingredients that bulk up the food content with little or no nutritional value. Beet pulp, which is primarily sugar, is one such substance; another is soybean meal, a leftover from the removal of most of the good oil from the bean. Sugar by-products, the inedible portions from the preparation and packaging of sugar-based food products such as candy, add calories and make food more palatable. Ground nut shells are another ingredient with questionable nutritional value.

Ingredients on labels can often be split listed, as in "meat by-products, ground corn, brewer's rice, corn meal." In this example, the main ingredient turns out to be corn because it's twice the amount of the first ingredient listed. Fats are not left out since they taste good, but the source of fat in pet food is usually restaurant grease, again unfit for humans but allowed for pets.

Once you begin to read labels, you will notice a long list of additional substances; these may be vitamins, minerals, or just additives. If vitamins and minerals are included, the manufacturer often adds an excess amount called "overage" to compensate for vitamin destruction during processing and to cover the shelf life of the product. An inordinate amount of some vitamins and minerals can cause serious illness or even death. There are lawsuits pending against companies for injuring or killing pets through excess quantities of these nutrients. Almost all pet food is loaded with preservatives, artificial flavors, and food dyes to turn gray food pink or red, giving it a "fresh" look. Preservatives ensure an endless shelf life, leading to rancidity; they are extremely toxic, even cancer causing. The most common are BHA, BHT, and ethoxyquin. Six types of waxes are approved for use on produce. Some of these are the same waxes used on automobiles, floors, and furniture: palm oil, shellac, paraffin, and synthetic resins.

To add the ultimate insult to the mix, the drug that is commonly used to euthanize dogs and cats, sodium pentobarbital (a barbiturate), is able to withstand the heat of rendering and thus finds its way into commercial pet food. The presence of pentobarbital has been detected in many lines of commercial pet food; any pet that eats this in foods on a daily basis for many years can develop life-threatening liver problems while building up a resistance to a drug that might be necessary should the pet need to be euthanized.

The best answer to the question of what to feed your pet is to home cook. With home cooking, you have the ability to make the best choices, use the best sources of food, and then supplement these with the appropriate amount of vitamins, minerals, herbs, and other phytonutrients. A home-cooked diet needs to take into consideration the age of the pet and should be adjusted periodically as your pet grows and ages. Different choices in nutrients can support your pet as he passes through different stages of his life. One size does not fit all, however. A supplement, for example, that seems to be helping the pet of a friend may not work the same way for your pet. A comprehensive nutritional program should be tailored to your pet's needs, taking into account his genetic and metabolic makeup, history, family background, lifestyle, and home environment. A working dog needs support that a dog of leisure does not; a cat in organ failure needs support that a healthy cat does not. The breed of the dog can point to possible problems that you can ward off with diet and phytonutrients.

You will find that you do have control over many issues that come up during the course of your pet's life. Cooking for your dog is empowering. The recipes in appendix B can help start you on a good support program. Try them.

5

INFLAMMATION AND CANCER

The body has evolved a great alarm system called inflammation. When it senses danger, it sets in motion a sequence of events designed to contain the danger. Inflammation can be triggered by the immune system; the cells of this system are always on high alert, and if some danger is encountered, they release message chemicals that lead to inflammation. The nervous system can trigger inflammation via sensory fibers running throughout the body. The nerves in the skin, the linings of the airways, the gastrointestinal tract, and the urogenital tract are especially vulnerable to traumatic stress, and when one of these systems is triggered, it releases chemicals that start the inflammatory process.

If cellular change can spark the fire of malignancy, inflammation is often the fuel that keeps the fire going. Inflammation is both an initiator and a promoter of cancer; there's been evidence of its role in this regard for two decades. Any disease that ends in -itis can be a harbinger of worse things to come. Once inflammation begins, it sets off a series of physiologic reactions. The process feeds on itself and becomes more and more difficult to turn off. "The world's most common cancers . . . have all been linked to inflammation."[1]

Inflammation should be seen as a whole-body issue, one with widespread effects; it should not be dismissed as merely a local phenomenon, the way someone might say, "Oh, that's just a painful joint." Inflammation in one part of the body will affect the chemistry in other parts as well. Inflammatory diseases are very common and insidious in humans and pets. Inflammation underlies asthma, irritable bowel syndrome, allergies, eczema, arthritis, high blood pressure, heart disease, and high cholesterol levels in humans and pets—to name only a few of the chronic problems many pets and people deal with. Some researchers argue that it is a factor in almost every disease state.

What was once thought to be a relatively simple body function turns out to be extraordinarily complex. Something as simple as banging a leg against a piece of furniture sets in motion a cascade of effects. Immediately, the body senses trauma and releases several different chemicals that start the inflammation process. Blood vessels open wider; the small vessels called capillaries leak fluid into the bloodstream and body tissues. A bump may occur from all this fluid. Immune cells move in, and more and more cells become involved. Intense cellular activity gets stirred up. And this is only for a simple trauma. Imagine what happens when the body is invaded by a virus, for example. How complex is that process?

Research has identified triggers, food being one of them, that promote inflammation; research has also identified anti-inflammatory agents, and food is one of them as well. If the boundaries of medical specialization are put aside, patterns begin to appear. A specific disease can often be related to many other diseases. The inflammatory connection reminds us that we must care for the whole body, not just the individual parts. Do we need to worry about inflammation? Of course. Our pets will experience one or more major inflammation-related diseases in their lives, such as arthritis, irritable bowel, or gum disease.

Chronic inflammation works to promote cancer at all stages of development; the longer the inflammation lasts, the higher the risk of cancer. Among the factors with the strongest links to cancer are infection and irritation in addition to inflammation. Bladder cancer is more common in those who have chronic or recurrent urinary tract infections. One study found that having three or more urinary tract infections doubles a person's risk of later developing bladder cancer. Hepatitis viruses can be linked to liver cancer. Epstein-Barr virus is linked to lymphoma.[2]

Mechanical or chemical irritation causes erosion inside the body. Where there is erosion, there will be inflammation attempting to fix the injured area. When the esophagus is repeatedly burned by digestive chemicals (as in the case of gastroesophageal reflux disease), the chemical irritation can lead to cancer. Kidney stones are a form of mechanical irritation of delicate body tissue that can also lead to inflammation. And inflammation left untreated or poorly treated for a long time can increase the risk of cancer; in the case of ulcerative colitis, for example, the risk of later colon cancer increases by five to seven times.

There are early triggers to sustained inflammation. Excess weight is one. Fat excretes pro-inflammatory chemicals and may tip the balance to increased risk of inflammation-related disorders. Getting some weight off of your cat or dog lowers the levels of inflammation and risk. The inflammatory chemical interleukin-6 plays a major role in many diseases, especially those pertaining to aging. In a healthy body, IL-6 levels are barely detected. With aging, IL-6 levels increase and are implicated in the loss of muscle mass and strength, cognitive decline, loss of bone mass, inflamed joints, and weakened heart muscle—explaining much of what happens with aging. Calorie restriction lowers the body's metabolic rate; consequently, fewer free radicals are made, and blood levels of IL-6 are reduced.

WHAT FOOD CAN DO TO HELP
REDUCE INFLAMMATION

The kind of food your pet eats is just as important as how much he eats. A diet consisting largely of meat, especially red meat, is a top inflammation trigger. One option is to eliminate beef from his diet, then, after a few weeks, eliminate another type of meat. Give your pet a vegetarian day once a week. If you are concerned about providing sufficient protein, substitute soy products, eggs, or other options, such as cottage or ricotta cheese, for a part of the meat portion.

You can expand his diet with fish. Oils from fish work at reducing inflammation and suppressing inflammatory chemicals. Fish oil has been shown to reduce the pain of inflammation as well as the risks of inflammation, such as a heart attack or stroke. The omega-3 essential fatty acids are the nutrients that provide this protection. (More on these shortly.) The highest concentrations of omega-3, meanwhile, can be found in mackerel, salmon, bluefish, anchovies, herring, trout, sardines, and mullet. Keep in mind that many types of fish now contain an unhealthy amount of methylmercury, a toxic carcinogen. Fish with the lowest levels of methylmercury are shrimp, salmon, pollack, mussels, scallops, and sole. Salmon is a good choice; not only is it low in toxicity, but it is high in omega-3 oils. Cats and dogs do enjoy salmon. Try to buy wild fish; the farm-raised kind is, for the most part, produced in the Pacific Rim countries in highly polluted water tanks, then cleaned with toxic chemicals before being shipped overseas to us.

What you feed your pet affects his body; food really is our most valuable tool for maintaining inflammation balance. With every meal, we have the option of increasing or decreasing inflammation. A mountain of research has made clear that eating lots of fruits and vegetables reduces the risk of many types of cancers. One study in the British medical journal *Lancet* showed that eating just one and a half servings of fruits or vegetables every day for six months reduced inflammation and increased the body's antioxidants.[3] What it comes down to is one salad, one apple, or one handful of raisins (or one grapefruit or one glass of orange juice for humans) that gives that extra one and a half serving.

What makes fruits and vegetables so beneficial? It is the compounds in plant food called phytochemicals that are so valuable as anti-inflammatory agents. In studies of animals fed with extracts of strawberry, blueberry, or spinach, not only were many age-related learning and memory deficits prevented, but they were actually reversed. Phytochemicals are available in their original packaging: the piece of fruit and the vegetable. Each and every fruit and vegetable has its own set of phytochemicals; good health depends on acquiring a full complement.

Flavonoid-rich vegetables and fruits are as good as corticosteroids, ibuprofen, and aspirin at inhibiting inflammatory enzymes (such as COX-2, TNF-alpha, and IL-8). The strategy is as follows: one cup of cooked broccoli, spinach, zucchini, or sweet potatoes added to one-half cup of fresh, uncooked raspberries, blueberries, blackberries, strawberries, or tomatoes or to one-half cup of fruits, such as apples, apricots, cantaloupe, or cranberries, with some parsley. Among the top inflammation-fighting foods are the cruciferous vegetables (kale, broccoli, Brussels sprouts, and so on), leafy green vegetables, citrus fruit, berries, and food rich in beta-carotene (those with dark orange colors). Don't get too caught up in servings. If you need to count, a serving is usually one item, such as half an apple for a medium-size to large dog, half a banana for a medium-size to large dog, and lesser portions for a small dog. A half cup of lightly cooked vegetables or a cup of uncooked leafy greens is a good serving for most dogs. A cat can eat about a quarter of a cup of vegetables a day, half in one meal and half in another. Use your hand; the amount you scoop up in the palm of your hand is a good serving for the average dog.

Preparation is just as important as selection. Avoid gumming up the proteins and carbohydrates and creating an abundance of highly inflammatory compounds by deep-frying or charcoal charring; instead stir-fry, poach, steam, stew, or boil. And since so little of the vast amount of produce we import is inspected by the Food and Drug Administration, try to buy organically grown fruits, vegetables, grains, and proteins.

As I noted earlier, contrary to popular myth, the body does need fat. It must be the right kind, however. The fats called essential fatty acids (EFAs) are in the necessary category. Every living cell needs EFAs; skin, hair, joints, arteries, heart, brain, glands, sperm, and nerve cells are dependent on having enough EFAs to keep them healthy. Since EFAs cannot be made by the body yet are "essential" to overall health, they must be obtained through food or supplements.

There are three groups of EFAs: omega-3 fatty acids, omega-6 fatty acids, and omega-9 fatty acids. Being unsaturated, these fats remain fluid. (For example, vegetable oils are unsaturated and fluid, while butter is saturated and solid at room temperature.) As part of the cell membrane structure, EFAs form a kind of barrier preventing foreign and toxic material from entering cells while keeping nutrients and genetic material inside.

A cell membrane is composed primarily of a two-layer construction. The outer layer is in contact with aqueous media around and within the cell; the inner layer has no contact with the fluid that surrounds it. This arrangement makes the cell membrane waterproof and unable to disintegrate into the fluid area while able to admit passage of both fat- and water-soluble molecules into the cells. If EFAs are deficient, destructive changes in the cell membranes can lead to poor metabolism and less energy both on the cell level and in the body in general.

An EFA deficiency is especially problematic for the brain. EFAs constitute one-half of all brain tissue. So important are EFAs to the brain that they are allowed to cross the blood–brain barrier. The function of this barrier is to stop most chemicals from getting into the brain and harming it. But EFAs are so vital that the barrier allows them to penetrate the brain rapidly and become incorporated into brain fats.

Omega-3 is by far the most important member of this family and the one most likely to be deficient in humans and dogs. Humans evolved on a diet that contained equal amounts of omega-3 and omega-6 fatty acids. About 100 years ago, the food supply changed; we began using hydrogenated (saturated) oils, which reduced the oil's omega-3 content. At the same time, the domestic livestock industry began to use feed grains, which are rich in omega-6 and low in omega-3 content. As a result, our diets are now at a ratio of 20 to 25 parts omega-6 to one part omega-3. The ratio should be one to one. Our diets and those of our dogs are now too high in omega-6, which may be a contributing factor in the rise of disease. A commercially prepared dog food has a high grain content and a high saturated fat content from animal products and by-products. We can assume that they face the same problem of too little omega-3 in the diet and too much omega-6. Japanese studies show that a diet rich in vegetables, fruit, soy products, and fish is one of the best and easiest solutions to an overconsumption of omega-6 fatty acids.

The reason that omega-3 is so much more important than omega-6 or -9 in the diet is because omega-3 is both an anticancer agent and an anti-inflammatory agent. This EFA inhibits tumor cell proliferation by slowing or delaying the development of cancer metastasis. There appears to be more than one way by which omega-3 may help to prevent the initiation and progression of tumors. Omega-3 is cytotoxic (deadly) to neoplastic (abnormal) cells. Increasing the availability of omega-3 will, in turn, increase cancer cell membrane fluidity; excessive increases in fluidity can cause cell death. This EFA effect on tumor cell membranes can be useful if a dog is undergoing chemotherapy. Omega-3 will increase the capacity for drug transport across the membrane. Studies show that omega-3 enhances the uptake of cytotoxic drugs (chemotherapy agents) into tumor cells.[4]

Omega-3 fatty acid can keep high levels of inflammation from developing; if there are already problems with inflammation, it can lessen their severity. Omega-3 is important in any course of treatment dealing with inflammatory issues: heart disease, connective tissue problems, dysplasia, all types of arthritis, diabetes, skin rashes, and allergies. In autoimmune diseases, omega-3 needs to be added in order to reduce inflammation.

Fish oils have proven to be the best source of omega-3. In one European study of 11,000 people who suffered heart attacks, half received a daily dose of fish oil at 1,000 milligrams and the other half a placebo. At the end of three months, more of those who received the fish oil supplements were alive than were those on the placebo. There was a 41 percent reduction in sudden death as well. At the end of three and a half years, the group taking fish oils had a 45 percent lower rate of fatalities. This effect was probably due in part to omega-3's ability to consistently prevent platelet aggregation and alter cholesterol levels.[5] Effective doses range all over the scale. In humans, 2 to 4 grams per day inhibits platelet aggregation, 4 grams suppresses inflammation, and 4 to 24 grams lowers plasma lipids. The effects become apparent within four weeks of administration. Dogs benefit from 1 gram per day regardless of size. However, a large dog will probably do better on 2 grams per day.

Omega-3 is made up of a series of acids. From canola and soybean oils, we can obtain alpha-linolenic acid; from walnut oil, we get stearidonic acid; and from cold-water, fatty fish, we get eicosatetraenoic (ETA) and eicosapentaenoic (EPA) acids. Of all these, the last two acids are the most important. Among their protective jobs are scavenging free radicals, inhibiting tumor cell access to blood circulation, inhibiting collagenases (a family of enzymes that eat up the collagen in connective tissue, causing joint degradation), and inhibiting plasmin, which degrades fibrin in the blood and in the components of a cell's matrix. Fish oils have the potential to inhibit cancer proliferation and progression, to promote the suicide (apoptosis) of cancer cells, and to induce differentiation in cancer cells (causing them to revert back to normal). Improved immune response and prolonged survival have also been documented in cancer patients supplemented with fish oils.

The omega-6 series comes from grains; it includes linolenic acids from most vegetable oils, nuts, and seeds; gamma-linolenic acids from evening primrose, borage, and black current seed oils; and di-homo-gamma-linolenic acids from animal fat sources, dairy, and eggs. Omega-6 is definitely beneficial when a dog is injured because of its clotting and blood vessel constriction effects.

The last member of the series is omega-9; the best-known source is cold-pressed olive oil from an organic source. The oil can be drizzled on your pet's food a few times a week. (Currently, we can add omega-5 and omega-7 to the -3, -6, and -9 series.)

Because of the body's inability to make these nutrients on its own, they must be obtained from food and supplementation. A lack of EFAs may affect a dog's recovery from a serious illness, especially cancer, for without them the body cannot mount an effective immune response. The problem in maintaining optimum levels is that most diets lose EFAs through processing heat and rancidity. Fat in food has a limited shelf life.

Further losses come from drugs and elevated toxins in our air, water, and food. High temperatures, such as in frying, destroy the EFA content in fish. The commercial dog food process damages most EFA nutrients that may once have been present. Dog food manufacturers often use hydrogenated oil (saturated solid fats), which, when heated to a very high temperature, as they typically are during processing, converts to a trans-fatty acid. These molecules have an unusual shape, causing interference with normal cell processes.

EFAs given over time must be accompanied by vitamin E to prevent an E deficiency, and, in turn, vitamin E keeps these polyunsaturated fats from turning rancid in the body and becoming free radicals. EFAs need the help of other nutrients, such as magnesium, selenium, and zinc; vitamin A; beta-carotene; and the B vitamins. When fish is your source of omega-3, be sure to choose salmon, herring, bluefish, tuna, sardines, or mackerel, which come from the cleanest waters of the world, to ensure noncontamination from mercury, PCBs, and other toxins. Buy the wild variety. Make sure that all EFAs are stored away from heat and light. You can freeze them if necessary, though, like all food sources, they're best fresh.

You can check to see if your dog may be deficient in EFAs by looking for symptoms of increased allergies, dry hair and skin, brittle nails, acne, eczema, rashes, or tiny lumps on the skin. If your dog has arthritis, an autoimmune problem, cardiovascular disease, high cholesterol, or cancer or appears to have lost his alertness or is aging, he needs EFAs.

A growing body of research links cancer initiation, promotion, progression, angiogenesis, and metastasis to inflammatory events. In other words, every aspect of cancer from beginning to end has an inflammation component. Anti-inflammatory agents reduce the invasiveness of cancer cell lines. Adequate control of inflammatory pathways must address multiple aspects of the inflammatory process. Using natural, nontoxic, anti-inflammatory strategies in a comprehensive approach is multifaceted.

Create a comprehensive protocol first through restricting animal-based foods—meat, dairy, and poultry—and substituting skinless, free-range poultry in moderation. Next, substantially increase dietary sources of omega-3, particularly EPA—available from cold-water fish and fish oil supplements (add fish from two to five times a week). Limit the intake of plant-source omega-6 (the ratio target should be one to one) to prevent enzyme competition. Begin to increase dietary antioxidants—deeply pigmented fruits and vegetables—to reduce oxidative stress. Eliminate saturated, hydrogenated, and trans-fatty acids; simple sugars; and refined carbohydrates from your pet's diet: processed biscuits, treats, and so on. Add zinc, magnesium, and vitamins E, C, and B complex—all coenzymes for metabolizing omega-3. If your pet's cholesterol levels are high, reduce them through nutrients such as herbs. And provide several anti-inflammatory botanical agents, such as enzymes, to modulate the inflammatory processes. Choices of agents should be based on their ability to provide multiple and synergistic actions. There'll be more on this in the next chapter.

The changes you make in your pet's diet will help reduce the risk of many problems. Food is one of our most valuable tools for maintaining inflammation balance.

6

ADD AMINO ACIDS AND ENZYMES

AMINO ACIDS

Not many substances are as important to cells as these amino acid proteins; they play a role in the work of enzymes, hormones, and genes—in fact, in every system in the body.

There are two distinct categories: those that must be obtained from diet, called essential amino acids, and those that are manufactured by the body or that are by-products of other amino acids, called nonessential amino acids. The fact that nonessential amino acids are termed nonessential doesn't mean that they are not necessary, only that they need not be obtained through diet because the body can manufacture them.

To understand how important amino acids are, let's follow the trail of one—glutamine—as it is used by the body. Glutamine is in great demand in the intestinal tract because it prevents the intestinal barrier wall from becoming compromised and allowing organisms such as undigested proteins and toxins to transfer across the barrier into the abdomen, where they can wreak all kinds of havoc. This is where autoimmune diseases begin and diseases such as leaky gut syndrome cause a lifetime of chronic illness.

Glutamine is also in high demand as the dominant amino acid in blood serum and cerebrospinal fluid. It is the only amino acid that is allowed easy passage through the blood–brain barrier and into the brain cavity. (The body has a protective roadblock in the blood–brain barrier. This barrier prevents many toxic substances from the rest of the body from entering the brain yet allows necessary chemicals through.) In the brain, glutamine couples with glucose to supply fuel to brain cells.

Glutamine serves as a major ammonia detoxification system in the form of glutamic acid, facilitating the brain's ability to rid itself not only of excess ammonia buildup but also of bacteria stemming from other forms of poisoning. This amino acid should be added to any treatment plan involving cancer work since one sequela of conventional treatment is toxic overload to the brain as well as other parts of the body.

Glutamine is vital to the nervous system. It produces and helps in the utilization of neurotransmitters, those little chemical messengers that travel back and forth between nerve endings. Most of the major neurotransmitters—serotonin, acetylcholine, dopamine, norepinephrine, and tryptophan—depend on glutamine's being available in the brain. It is a precursor of gamma-aminobutyric acid (GABA), a calming type of neurotransmitter that is often recommended as part of the treatment for epilepsy and hyperactivity.

Once we leave the brain and get to the body proper, we discover that glutamine is a component of the glucose tolerance factor chromium, which is needed to synthesize cholesterol, fats, proteins, and carbohydrates for energy and to keep stable blood sugar levels through insulin utilization. Researchers estimate that because the average American diet is chromium deficient (only one in 10 of us has an adequate amount of chromium for normal insulin levels), two out of every three of us are prehyperglycemic, hyperglycemic, or diabetic.

Glutamine is an important amino acid for cancer treatment because it can make tumor cells more sensitive to radiation or chemotherapy agents. With the help of glutamine, these therapies are more likely to succeed while the patient experiences less toxicity to the gut, more normal levels of red and white blood cells, a lower likelihood of sepsis, and a better chance of survival.

But all amino acids are important. There are 26 known amino acids, combining in many ways to create the hundreds of different types of proteins that make up our bodies. Each amino acid has specific functions, so for therapeutic purposes, it's wise to supplement with a full amino acid complex, which includes essential and nonessential types. This ensures that there are adequate amounts of all the amino acids in the body. A good rule to follow is to back up the individual amino acid being prescribed with a complex of them for about two months and then discontinue the complex for two months. Keep the dosage under 1,000 milligrams and always include vitamins B and C in the program to enhance absorption. When using amino acids as therapy, you'll want to choose according to function. Let's look at these super-helpers.

The amino acids that are sulfur derivatives—methionine, cystine, glutathione, thionine, cysteine, glutamic acid, taurine, and glycine—have one important function in common: they detoxify heavy metals, such as lead, cadmium, mercury, and aluminum and overloads of copper and iron. In addition, they are free radical scavengers. Glutathione is an amino acid that contains cysteine, glycine, and glutamic acid—three amino acids in one—and because of its sulfur content provides antioxidant activity. Glutathione converts hydrogen peroxide (a dangerous free radical) into water. It assists the liver in metabolizing drugs and protects the integrity of red blood cells. It deactivates free radicals from fats that can suppress the immune system as well as being carcinogenic and mutagenic. Glutathione may also help prevent cancer. Harvard Medical School studies have shown that glutathione has the ability to enhance a cell's immune protective status by preventing impairment of phagocytes, the white blood cells that destroy foreign matter and harmful bacteria.[1] There seems to be a special role for this amino acid in reducing liver tumors. In one study, the use of glutathione caused partial or complete remission in 81 percent of induced liver tumors.[2]

Choose inclusion of an amino acid to an anticancer treatment plan for its therapeutic use:

- Retarding tumors by enhancing immune functions: arginine, aspartic acid, carnitine, and serine
- Guarding against toxic buildup: alanine, aspartic acid, citruline, cysteine, cystine, glutamic acid, and glutamine
- Aiding in sugar and fat metabolism to increase stamina: arginine, aspartic acid, carnitine, citruline, glutamic acid, glycine, isoleucine, serine, and tyrosine
- Assisting the brain and nervous system in antiaging and slowing down degeneration: asparagine, aspartic acid, carnitine, cysteine, cystine, GABA, glutamic acid, glutamine, histidine, lysine, phenylalanine, taurine, tryptophan, and tyrosine

- Treating anemia: histidine
- Protecting against the negative effects of radiation exposure: cysteine, histidine, and tryptophan
- Treating virus-induced problems and rebuilding the myelin sheath on damaged nerves: histidine, lysine, and serine
- Rebuilding bone and tendon cells: arginine, cysteine, glutamine, glycine, leucine, phenylalanine, proline, taurine, threonine, and valine

The processes that the amino acids perform depend on bioavailability. An inadequate supply of even one amino acid can cause problems. All the amino acids must be present in the diet in order for all to be used. Many factors contribute to deficiencies: impaired absorption of food, infections, trauma, stress, drugs, age, and imbalances of the vitamins B and C. If a body becomes deficient, sooner or later some type of physical disorder will develop. Several amino acid deficiencies have been linked to iron deficiency, autoimmune problems, allergies, depression, impaired neurology, fatigue, impotence, schizophrenia, and senility.

When supplementing, be sure to give on an empty stomach so that there is no competition between amino acids in the supplement and in food. Supplemental amino acids come as an "L" form, or "levo" (Latin for "left"). These are the nutrients considered compatible with the body's biochemistry. The supplement will be labeled L-lysine, for example. Amino acids are nontoxic and can be used in long-term care and readily purchased in health supply stores.

ENZYMES

Most people think of enzymes (if they think of them at all) as necessary only if they have some kind of digestive problem. And, yes, it's true that people and dogs with digestive problems have benefited greatly from using enzyme supplements. But if that's all you think enzymes are good for, you don't know the half of it. Both how long a body lives and how fast it ages are directly related to the exhaustion of its enzymes' potential. In other words, having a full enzyme potential equates with a longer, healthier, and more vital life.

Enzymes are everywhere in our life: they make dough rise, they ripen cheese, they ferment foods, and they clean our clothes. In fact, the development of life would have been impossible without enzymes.

Scientists today know that up to 40,000 enzymes are involved in all the biological processes on earth. They are among the busiest molecules in the body. In fact, a single enzyme can spring into action up to 36 million times a minute.

There are two main groups of these tiny complex chains of proteins, and every enzyme performs a specific task. One group acts outside the cell and is responsible for gathering up food nutrients, metabolizing them, and transporting usable ones to the cell. The other group works inside the cell as a quality-control delivery system, allowing only the best standard nutrients to pass through the cell membrane.

A cell has no use for a bite of food. It's too big to be absorbed. Food, therefore, has to be broken down into its individual nutrients for the cell to use; this is done by enzymes. The breakdown begins in the mouth, where special digestive enzymes called amylase, which is contained in saliva, start the process The first task is to destroy any harmful substances in the food, such as bacteria. Then the enzymes separate the sugar and starch molecules from the food.

Next on the assembly line, the chewed food is delivered to the stomach. The stomach's gastric acid destroys the last remaining harmful substances—more bacteria and even viruses. This process destroys the amylase but leaves the pepsin enzymes to begin their work on proteins. At this point, the food leaves the stomach, reaches the duodenum, and meets a different set of enzymes produced by the pancreas and liver. The ingested food is now getting smaller and smaller until it reaches microscopic size. Intestinal enzymes process it into proteins, which in turn are split into their individual components: the amino acids and small molecules of carbohydrates. With the help of bile acids donated from the gallbladder, the fats and oils in food will be converted into usable nutrients. All these different nutrients are transported through the wall of the intestine into the blood and on to the cells. Essential vitamins and minerals provided by the food are transported throughout the body by enzyme activity. And the unusable remains of the food continue to the large intestine, where enzymes trigger the process of fermentation and eventual excretion.

Digestion is not an enzyme's sole reason to be. Enzymes are also crucial in enhancing the activity of the immune system. Protective linings in the mouth and nose are home to an enzyme—lysozyme—capable of dissolving intruders such as viruses, bacteria, fungi, and other pathogens from the environment. Inside the body, enzymes whip up other defense mechanisms:

the antibodies and, especially, the macrophages. When attacked, the antibodies stick to intruders relentlessly until these foreigners are destroyed by macrophage action. Armed with enzymes, macrophages can destroy intruders up to 10 times faster.

Enzymes cohabit and work in the body with the support of other biological substances. These helpers are coenzymes, usually vitamins, such as those in the B and C families, and minerals and trace elements, such as sodium, magnesium, iron, copper, zinc, manganese, and selenium. A coenzyme deficiency means that the enzymes will not be able to function properly. For example, enzymes need the cooperation of the B vitamins to maintain energy through amino acid (protein) breakdown as well as fat and carbohydrate breakdown, the formation of hemoglobin (red blood cells), and maintaining nervous system integrity.

Coenzymes are highly sensitive and have dangerous enemies. The food sources where these helpers are found can lose up to 60 percent of their potency during long journeys and extended stays in cupboards. Cooking destroys coenzymes; steaming or lightly cooking vegetables will help to retain 70 percent of the water-soluble coenzymes. Soaking and cooking vegetables in water destroys more than half of their valuable vitamins, and vitamins will not survive in prolonged food warming.

The environment also kills enzymes. Environmental poisons, such as carbon monoxide, mercury, lead, cadmium, copper compounds, and cyanide, obstruct enzyme activity. Copper pipes in a home will also kill enzymes. Exhaust fumes from a busy street will settle on produce at a farmer's market and destroy coenzymes. Medications, particularly antibiotics, laxatives, and painkillers, pose a threat to the body's vitamin and mineral balance. Even aging causes deficiencies; enzymes will show signs of wear and tear. They lose their strength, and it takes longer and longer for the body to produce replacements.

What may be the most important powers of enzymes are often overlooked: their ability to combat inflammation and autoimmune disease, prevent sports injuries and swelling, assist in the body's preparation for surgery, treat immune-complex illnesses, alleviate vein complaints, and prevent arteriosclerosis and cancer. The use of enzymes in this way is called "systemic enzyme therapy." "Systemic" means simply that the enzymes are distributed through the body via the bloodstream.

Therapy for conditions involving inflammation, such as joint, muscle, tendon, bone, and spine repair, will consist of combinations containing both animal-based and plant-based enzymes. Bromelain, papain, boswellia, hyaluronic acid, horse chestnut, and devil's claw are some of the ingredients you may find on the enzyme product label. The enzymes in this mixture reduce swelling by breaking down large protein molecules in the tissue and removing them. Less swelling leads to less pressure on the nerves, meaning less pain. Multienzyme preparations, even in high doses, can be taken over long periods of time with no side effects.[3]

Enzyme preparations are often in the form of coated tablets that are not easily dissolved by the stomach. Thus, the enzymes are able to reach the intestines, then the bloodstream, and eventually their place of work. Because many of the enzymes will be lost in transit, a preparation will contain many different enzymes in large doses. In these multienzyme preparations, all the enzymes are effective, so it's possible to treat a number of different ailments. Multienzyme preparations containing pancreatin, bromelain, trypsin, papain, and chymotrypsin are best because they have so many uses.

Every injury to the body initially results in swelling. This is caused by protein molecules that have broken off from the blood into the tissue. The goal of this action is to compress blood vessels so that the wound will not bleed indefinitely. Swelling causes pain because of compression on the surrounding nerve endings. At some point, the action has to be stopped so that healing will take place. It's enzymes that come to the rescue. Once enzymes are consumed, a wound will heal in a matter of days. Nutrients and oxygen will begin flooding the area, and waste products will be removed.

Inflammation is always a sure sign that something is wrong. It could mean that a pathogen has entered or that there is a defect in the tissue, such as in the case of a wound. Regardless of cause, the body's defensive measures begin to restore tissue to its normal healthy state as quickly as possible.

First, histamine is released; its role is to transport more blood to the area and activate the antibodies of the immune system. The inflamed area swells from the blood and becomes red on the outside and hot to the touch. Once again, here come the enzymes. They get busy removing dead tissue and waste products, breaking down the protein molecules responsible for the swelling, and quickening the healing process by bringing fresh nutrients to the area.

When swelling and inflammation continue unabated and the body's immune system malfunctions, attacking itself instead of the invading pathogens, the problem gets a bit more difficult to solve. Antibodies, instead of attaching themselves to an enemy, have attached themselves to body tissue;

they can be annihilated only by destroying this healthy tissue. Picture an immune system running riot, with macrophages constantly forming new immune complexes and lodging them in the tissues while the complementary part of the immune system continues to destroy them, along with more and more healthy tissue. Now you can understand how an organ is eventually overcome with severe inflammation, swelling, fever, and, ultimately, necrosis (death). (There'll be more detail on this in an upcoming chapter.)

Enzymes are incredibly useful, and if the body's life span is directly related to the exhaustion of its enzyme potential, how could you not be using them? But which enzymes should you use? Look for a mixture that contains several that digest protein, such as protease and papain; some for starch and carbohydrate digestion, such as amylase; cellulose to break down fiber cellulose into small units; lipase and bromelain to digest fats; and, finally, lactase to aid in the digestion of dairy products. Good enzyme products will also include coenzyme factors: minerals, algae (spirulina and chlorella), and ionic minerals. Another ingredient you may add yourself is betaine HCL—especially good for the older body, which does not always produce enough stomach acid.

Enzyme supplements for digestion should be taken with a meal. Betaine is best taken as a separate supplement about a half hour after eating. Of course, enzyme therapy needs to be complemented with good eating habits. Fresh fruits, vegetables, nuts, and seeds can provide plant enzymes that will predigest the food. Whole, unprocessed food with plenty of raw ingredients included offers the most benefit. This diet will provide not only plant enzymes but the necessary coenzymes as well.

But the most important use of enzymes lies in their use as systemic enzyme therapy. This is the subject of a great deal of research, especially in Europe. The consensus among scientists is that the depletion of plant enzymes leads to a host of chronic diseases that could, at least in part, be prevented if the body had the enzymes it needed. Enzyme deficiencies are not typically something medical or laypeople are aware of because they take so long to manifest. By the time there are signs of a deficiency, the body is in a state of exhaustion.

Processing and cooking destroy enzymes in food; this means that the food entering our stomachs is severely enzyme and coenzyme deficient. Studies show that including more raw foods in your pet's diet could possibly allow him to live 30 percent longer than with a processed, cooked diet devoid of enzymes.

Systemic enzyme therapy is the use of pancreatic enzymes that are taken between meals and not needed for digesting food; they make their way into the bloodstream and aid in the elimination of what are called "circulating complexes." If too many circulating complexes accumulate, the kidneys cannot excrete them, meaning that they accumulate in soft tissue, causing inflammation. This is an unnecessary stressor on the immune system that results in continuous work on the part of the system as well as the initiation of abnormal cells. Enzymes taken between meals will digest foreign proteins and infecting organisms, such as viruses, scar tissue, and the products of inflammation. For this reason, pancreatic enzymes or systemic enzyme therapy can be useful in those suffering from chronic illnesses and are recommended prior to surgery. Interestingly enough, because viruses have a protein coat, enzymes are able to start reactions that can digest this protective layer.

Pancreatic enzymes can help in the treatment of cancer. They do this by exposing antigens on the surface of cancer cells. Once these antigens are recognized as foreign, they become targets for the major anticancer agents: the T-cells, the tumor necrosis factor cells, and the natural killer cells. The enzymes can also remove the sticky coating found on tumor cells, reducing the risk of a tumor adhering to other areas of the body. And pancreatic enzymes can enter cancer cells during their reproductive phase. Together with the help of vitamin A, the destructive effect is enhanced, causing tumors to dissolve.

All in all, enzymes equal life. By supplementing with enzymes, you will notice a significant reduction in indigestion problems that your pet may have, relief from gas and bloating, diminished food allergies, and an increase in energy. Knowing this, how could you not use them and insist that everyone—human or animal—you know and love use them every time they eat?

In the words of Dr. Edward Howell, a pioneer researcher on the benefits of enzymes, "It's just as if you inherited a certain amount of money and didn't save any. If you spend it all, you won't have any more money in the bank. It's the same with enzymes. You inherit a certain enzyme potential, and it must last a lifetime."[4]

Enzymes are particularly useful as indicators as to the nature and progress of a medical problem and are listed in what is called a combined blood count that your veterinarian uses. These enzymes are characterized as follows:

- *Alkaline phosphatase:* Alkaline phosphatase is naturally occurring in bones, liver, bile ducts, and the lining of the small intestine. Increased enzyme activity points to such problems as a tumor's metastasizing to the bones or a hyperfunctioning of the parathyroid gland. An elevation seen in a lab analysis is very often a sign that the liver and/or bile ducts are beginning to develop serious problems.
- *Alpha amylase:* Raised levels of this enzyme could indicate a possible problem in the pancreas, where it is produced. Since the enzyme breaks down sugars and starches, elevated levels may mean that the pancreas is inflamed or that the exit ducts are defective.
- *Angiotensin I converting enzyme:* This enzyme regulates blood pressure and indicates negative changes in the system.
- *Cholinesterase:* This enzyme, if reduced dramatically, indicates liver cell damage and cirrhosis. The damage could relate to overexposure to pesticides, insecticides, or other environmental toxins.
- *Creatine kinase:* This enzyme rises dramatically after a heart attack. It is a lifesaving indicator in that it can show that a heart attack has taken place. Creatine kinase is also involved in muscular and skeletal areas, and a raised level could also be the result of muscular injuries and inflammation.
- *Gamma glutamyl transferase:* These enzymes are found in several organs, including the liver, kidneys, pancreas, spleen, and the small intestines. An elevated level would point to problems in these organs. In the liver, for example, high levels would indicate cirrhosis due to medications or a fatty liver.
- *Glutamate dehydrogenase:* Elevation of this enzyme indicates a serious liver problem. This enzyme would be elevated as a result of poisoning.

See the "Resources" section in this book for supplemental sources of amino acids and enzymes. Food sources of enzymes are plentiful. You can include in your pet's food plan pineapple, papaya, avocados, bananas, sprouts, seeds, and legumes. Vegetable sources are broccoli, Brussels sprouts, and cabbage. Eggs can be included as well.

7

NATURAL ANTICANCER AGENTS

VITAMINS

More than most people realize, nutrients play a huge role in cancer treatment and prevention. Refining, processing, preparing, and cooking can rob food of vital nutrients.

Farming practices have decreased the nutrient value in soil, and fertilizers can block the availability of vitamins and minerals in plants. Food additives further add to this lack of availability. Having cancer and going through conventional chemotherapy often have such a profound impact on a patient's nutritional status that, according to researchers reporting from the MD Anderson Hospital and Tumor Institute in Texas, malnutrition becomes a major cause of death: "Cancer and cancer chemotherapy often have such a profound impact on a patient's nutritional status that malnutrition becomes a major cause of morbidity and mortality."[1] Malnutrition can be turned around with food as well as supplements.

As a caring companion to your pet, you have probably considered supplementing him with a vitamin pill. Vitamins, by definition, are substances essential to the normal growth and functioning of the body. A shortage or lack of any one vitamin results in an immediate and measurable deficiency or disease condition. As we have learned more about them, we have come to realize how important vitamins A, B, C, D, and E are to health.

Vitamin deficiencies will produce measurable problems often within a short time. Deficiencies have been associated with cancer, heart disease, blood disorders, and other serious conditions. It appears that some of the best work vitamins do is keeping the total load of toxins down. Unfortunately, we don't know how much is too much when it comes to toxins.

It turns out that everyone, everywhere, now carries in their body a huge array of chemical contaminants. These accumulate in bones, fat, blood, and organs. Scientists studying pollutants call the phenomenon "chemical body burden," the total result of womb-to-tomb exposure to chemicals in food, water, and almost every common substance we use. No place, no one, and no animal is immune. Chemical contaminants cross borders, oceans, and continents and settle in and biomagnify themselves. In the United States, more than 80,000 industrial substances are registered for commercial purposes. About 10,000 of these chemicals are in everyday items, such as clothes, cleaning supplies, and furniture. Scientists are not yet able to tell us much about what this exposure might mean to us individually.

When we look outside the United States to other cultures and their rates of disease, we find some interesting information. The French, for example, have a high-fat diet loaded with sugar and would seem likely to have a higher rate of heart disease than Americans. But no, they are 2.5 times less likely to have cardiovascular problems than we are. Research credits whole, fresh foods, particularly flavonoid-rich food compounds providing vitamin P. Broccoli, celery, grapes, apples, and other nutritionally dense, whole foods in the French diet provide a protective effect in the bloodstream. The flavonoids keep the clumping together of blood cells to a minimum and prevent plaque buildup, heart disease, and stroke.[2]

In Japan, the smoking rate is twice that of the United States, yet the rate of lung cancer in that country is half the rate in the United States. The difference, again, is attributed to diet: daily intake of soy products, vegetables, fruits, and seaweeds. The nutrients in these food compounds protect healthy cells.[3] This protection has been demonstrated in more than 9,000 studies on whole foods.

Along with accumulated toxins, there is another common denominator linking many of our diseases. It is estimated that more than 60 chronic conditions, including advanced, rapid aging, are attributed to this one menace. It is the reason that we and our pets are unlikely to reach our full potential life span. It is free radicals.

Free radicals are the by-products of normal body metabolism. They are molecules that are missing an electron, making them unstable and, thus, constantly on the move to find a mate for that one single electron. They think nothing of robbing an electron from a normal cell, even though, in the process, they cause mutation in normal cells, possibly turning those cells cancerous. Indeed, cells are constantly being damaged by free radicals. Our health is directly related to the limitation of free radical production, and this limitation can take place only if the body has enough free radical scavengers.

The body's production of free radicals is constant, as is the body's vigilance in dealing with them. However, there are factors that cause more than the normal amount of free radical production: poor diet, prolonged nutritional deficiencies, stress, chronic disease, medicinal drugs, pollutants, and contaminated water—just about everything in our environment is a free radical promoter.

Chemotherapy usually involves the use of several antineoplastic (anticancer) drugs. The drugs in this category are toxic to cancer cells, but all of them are toxic to healthy cells as well. It's this toxicity that causes numerous side effects. One major problem in the process of killing off unhealthy cells is the creation of oxidative damage, another term for free radicals.

Let's look more closely at the problems that free radicals cause. Fifty years ago, Dr. Denham Harmon, a medical researcher and practitioner, discovered that free radical reactions could be responsible for the progressive deterioration that typically accompanies the aging process. Harmon theorized that reducing free radical damage was one very important solution to disease and aging. This is the role of antioxidants.

Antioxidants counter the action of free radicals by attaching to them and providing their missing electron. There is no single antioxidant that protects all parts of the body; rather, the individual antioxidants are distinguished in part by the areas of the body in which they are the most effective. Those that protect the eyes from free radical damage would not be as effective for the brain or the heart. This is why it is so important to consume a variety of foods and supplements that have many different antioxidants.

Back in 1954 and for many more decades, Harmon's conclusions were discounted by other scientists who thought that the free radical theory was too simple to account for something as complex as aging. One scientist, however, was intrigued. Dr. Richard Passwater entered into an informal collaboration with Harmon that would turn out to be both long and extremely fruitful. Passwater discovered that antioxidants worked and that they worked synergistically; when given in combinations, antioxidants were more potent than when used individually. For example, Harmon discovered that any life span could be increased by a tiny bit (up to 5 percent) with small amounts of vitamin E taken on a regular basis. When Passwater began giving his research subjects vitamin C in addition to vitamin E, he found that life spans increased by a startling 20 to 25 percent.

The body makes many of its own antioxidants; among these are enzymes, coenzymes, and sulfur-containing chemicals. But the majority of antioxidants are introduced from outside the body: the amino acids, vitamins, minerals, and natural substances, such as flavonoids and carotenoids, and essential fatty acids, such as omega-3. Scientists now know that free radical damage plays a role in more than 200 diseases. Harmon believed that antioxidant nutrients were the heart of medicine.

It is generally recognized in alternative medical circles that antioxidants are underutilized. As more and more attention is paid to them, we hear the same questions: which ones should be used, for what purpose, for how long, at what dosages, in what delivery strategy, and with what frequency? Eating a plant-based diet will give you most of the important antioxidants: vitamin C, beta-carotene, vitamin E, and many cancer-fighting phytochemicals (nutrients from plants). These antioxidants are considered the best protection against aging and environment-related diseases. Antioxidants mop up the toxic chemicals of everyday living and the by-products of daily body chemistry activities.

The amazing thing about these supplements is the many roles they play in the body: they moderate and regulate chemical reactions, they heal sick organs and rejuvenate health, they empower the body to fight off potentially dangerous invaders, and they keep abnormal changes to a minimum. They are not toxic, nor do they have side effects, and they can be taken on an indefinite basis.

Some oncologists believe that patients undergoing chemotherapy should avoid supplementing with antioxidants. The idea is that an antioxidant may interfere with the oxidative damage to cancer cells intentionally caused by chemotherapy drugs. However, this theory does not hold up under the scrutiny of scientific research. A look at all the studies clearly shows that antioxidants need not be avoided for fear that they will interfere with chemotherapy. Reports have repeatedly concluded that there is much to gain

in protection and support from adding supplements to an anticancer protocol. In fact, reversing its long-held stance on the value of supplements, the
Journal of the American Medical Association recommends that all adults
take a multivitamin daily.

A good nutrition program uses food compounds for their unique ad-
vantages, primarily the way they break down into vitamins, minerals,
amino acids, enzymes, and other nutrients. Almost all food compounds
provide potent antioxidants (anti–free radical scavengers). Although the
body produces many different antioxidants, if there is an overload of free
radicals, production can't keep up with the need. This situation puts all
body systems at risk for irreversible damage. This is especially true for
cells. If free radical damage is persistently high, the result is disease
and accelerated aging. Food compounds and whole-food vitamins can
step in as sponges, soaking up excess free radicals, but food-compound
activity comes from incorporating a variety and an abundance of these
substances into the diet.

Whole foods and food-compound vitamins protect the body's chemical
balances. They are partly responsible for cellular and metabolic equilib-
rium within cell structure and between cells and their environments. They
enable cells to access more energy through the efficient use of oxygen.
Food-compound vitamins balance blood pressure and water metabolism
and regulate body temperature and cholesterol levels. They increase the
body's resistance to the adverse effects of stress by supporting adrenal
gland functions. Since different food compounds exhibit strong bonds to
specific organs, a diet must have a complete range of these compounds. If
there is only one big idea that has come out of the research done on food
compounds and food-compound vitamins, it is that while there is considerable overlap among these nutrients, humans and animals need to eat a
"rainbow" of them.

Let's look at one family group—the carotenoids—to get a picture of
what actually occurs with food compounds and vitamins. Carotenoids are
a class of nutrients that are made of fat-soluble pigments of yellow, red,
orange, and green. There are more than 500 carotenoids found in nature;
about 50 of them can be converted into a vitamin A–like nutrient. There
is no one vitamin A; carotenoids are complexes of vitamin A, many times
acting as precursors to the formation of vitamin A in the body.

Within the carotenoids are subclasses. Best known among these are the
carotenes, beta-carotene being one; within that group is lycopene. This

nutrient is found in tomatoes and is tied to a reduced risk of prostate and lung cancer as well as a variety of digestive cancers. Another subclass, the xanthophylls, gives us lutein and zeaxanthin; lutein comes from dark, leafy greens, such as broccoli, and zeaxanthin is found in other dark, leafy greens, such as kale and spinach. These two carotenes are effective in protecting cells in the eyes from free radical damage. Two other subclasses are the limonoids, including limonene, and phytosterols, including perillyl alcohol, both of interest as antitumor agents. This may seem a bit complicated, but the main idea is to use a variety of carotene compounds to secure the protection you're looking for. Load your plate and your pet's plate with vegetables, especially those having the brightest colors—oranges, yellows, and reds—and the deepest, darkest greens and purples.

The best supplements are those that are made from food. This gives the supplement a broader spectrum of nutrients than a regular natural vitamin—and definitely more than a synthetic vitamin—offers. The more nutrients you get, the greater the potential for better results. Food-formed and food-compound vitamins have a high rate of utilization by the body. They inherently contain vital food factors working as precursors, enhancers, and supporters of the vitamin; these are necessary for nutrient delivery and bioavailability. Food-compound vitamins give the body exactly what it needs.

Returning to vitamin A, this vitamin works better with the assistance of carotenoids in foods eaten along with it. Vitamin C works better with citrus foods and other foods that contain compounds called flavonoids. Vitamin E can be bought in the synthetic or the natural form. Vitamin E found in foods has seven complementary food compounds or relatives that, when combined, result in higher nutrient delivery to the body; they're even more effective than natural vitamin E by itself and superior to the synthetic form.

Vitamins made from food and food compounds cost more, but they are the most cost-effective option because they offer a high potency level. One doesn't need the megadoses required by synthetic vitamins. It's important to use your money wisely. How do you know if your multivitamin is the best that you can buy? Look at the supplement facts box on the back of the label. This information was added recently by the government to inform consumers about what is actually in the vitamin. First, you'll find the name—vitamin C, for example. To the right of this is the form, or type, of vitamin C. Usually, this is a chemical name showing that it is laboratory created; it has not been made from food and doesn't contain food compounds. Even though there may be pictures of oranges or the word "natural" on the label, there is no food involved. If the label refers to the product as "ascorbic acid," it is still a manufactured product. The structure of the vitamin is the same as that found in food, but it is an isolated nutrient. It works alone, and to get much benefit, you or your dog would have to take two, three, or more of these pills a day.

The information on the container of a vitamin bottle that has whole-food sources and is a food-compound vitamin would read "vitamin C and oranges"—not the picture but the food itself. Each supplement you buy should have a food supporting each vitamin on the label, stating something like "ascorbic acid, oranges compounded." Look further for the extraction number. It is usually listed as 4×, 5×, and so on, meaning that the food has been extracted to be equal to four or five times that of the raw food. "Broccoli extract 5:1" means that the broccoli has been extracted from real food to be five times more potent than the equal raw amount. You are getting five times the amount of nutrients from the broccoli than if you ate one raw serving. If the vitamin contains 50 milligrams of broccoli 5×, you are getting 250 milligrams of the wonderful nutrients broccoli provides.

Consider vitamins made from whole food and food compounds as health insurance. You and your pet will get the lipids, organic acids, polysaccharides, phenols, organosulfurs, amines, and terpenes—all seven classes of the food compounds necessary for health and all in one bottle. You will get the right absorption, the correct delivery mechanisms, and peak utilization of every nutrient you need. No other type of vitamin supplement can make this claim. Since the body needs all the help it can get to deal with the day-to-day chemicals it meets, these are the only vitamins you should consider using.

Many of the functions of vitamins are poorly understood; studies can end with confusing results since eating habits are complex and foods contain multiple micronutrients. (For example, vitamin P can have as many as 200 nutritional units called flavonoids.) However, a review of epidemiologic studies uniformly shows a definite therapeutic and preventive role for vitamins in cancer. Sources of bioactive components are the following:

Broccoli: Reduces oxidative stress and carcinogen metabolism
Berries: Reduce malignant transformation
Tomatoes: Reduce oxidative stress
Grapes: Provide anti-inflammatory benefits
Avocados: Reduce apoptosis

VITAMIN A

Data from experiments consistently highlight the ability of vitamin A and its precursors, the carotenoids, to protect against all cancer types. High levels of carotenes in the blood support differentiation of epithelial cells and are associated with a decreased risk of epithelial cancer (lung, esophageal, and mouth). One of the roles it plays is in promoting and regulating apoptosis, or the death of abnormal cells—the same role as chemotherapy agents.

Vitamin A is a natural antioxidant against smoke and other pollutants. The respiratory tract and eye tissues are constantly assaulted by air pollutants, and the amount of free radicals in these toxins is enormous. Vitamin A soaks up environmental free radicals; it repairs damage and boosts the immune system.

Vitamin A supplements change the type of immune response the body produces. Even a moderate amount of supplementation over a short period of time changes the way white blood cells respond. To identify and destroy abnormal cells, white blood cells must first distinguish them from normal cells. They do this through a protein called MHC class II. When a bad cell is found, the protein alerts the white cells, which then attack and remove the abnormal cell. If the white blood cells don't have enough of these proteins, the abnormal cells slip by. Vitamin A, in the form of carotenoids, increases the number of the MHC class II proteins, and immunity surveillance is thus enhanced.

One carotenoid, beta-carotene, helps make a chemical specific to fighting cancer called tumor necrosis factor alpha (TNF). Macrophages (members of the immune system) secrete TNF in an attempt to destroy cancer cells and other foreign cells. TNF also has a secondary effect, namely, mobilizing fat and protein energy stores for use, scientists believe, as energy sources for immune cells.

Vitamin A is found in two basic forms: retinols and carotenoids. Retinol is the form found in food sources such as cod liver oil, liver, egg yolks, and dairy products and is active immediately on digestion. Carotenoids are really provitamins converted into vitamin A by the liver. Their sources are foods from plants that are dark green, leafy vegetables (such as broccoli), red (such as tomatoes), and yellow-orange (such as squash).

A diet rich in vegetables and fruits filled with vitamin A provides fiber and antioxidant protection that is very important to the colon. Moreover, the incidence of breast cancer is related both to the intake of fruits and vegetables containing vitamin A and to the amount of vitamin A and carotenoids stored in fat tissue. Vitamin A and related carotenoid compounds actually help in gene transcription, that is, in the copying of genes when a new cell is formed. If there is enough vitamin A, the genes copy more accurately, meaning fewer mistakes and abnormal cells. Your pet may be a candidate for vitamin A supplementation if his levels of the vitamin have been reduced by exposure to air pollution (something just about all dogs, cats, and birds have in common). Other factors that diminish levels of the vitamin in the body are chronic health problems (cancer being one), recurrent infections, a diet high in fat, a fat or protein deficiency, or long-term use of analgesics, such as nonsteroidal anti-inflammatory drugs (NSAIDs) or steroid medications. A pet with renal failure will show extraordinarily low concentrations of the vitamin as well as all the other fat-soluble vitamins (vitamins D and E). It's almost impossible to overdose on this vitamin if it is obtained from dietary sources alone. In short, vitamin A and carotenoids minimize cell damage.

VITAMIN C

In its role as a powerful antioxidant, detoxifier, and healer, vitamin C is probably the nutrient most associated by the public with cancer prevention. This vitamin makes up a family consisting of itself and vitamin P, the bioflavonoids. One of its greatest benefits is that it fights the effects of pollution. Because our pets breathe air and drink water, the toxic products produced—the free radicals—are precursors to malignancies. Floating in the liquid of the cell, this vitamin neutralizes free radicals before they ever reach the membrane of the mitochondrial part of the cell. This protection reduces the amount of energy it takes for the mitochondria to fight oxidation and leaves more energy for the life of the cell.

Vitamin C is generous to the body, helping to boost other vitamins, particularly vitamins A and E. If a steady intake of the vitamin is maintained, it can recycle the fat-soluble vitamins.

Vitamin C is believed to inhibit carcinogenesis, or tumor growth, in several ways. First, this vitamin is necessary for the maintenance of the extracellular matrix; a growing tumor will begin to crowd out its neighbors unless vitamin C is present to inhibit tumor invasion. Vitamin C intake stimulates the increase of natural killer (NK) cell activity. NK cells are capable of killing a broad range of solid tumors, leukemic, and virus-infected cells. The vitamin is a natural antioxidant, capable of inhibiting cancer initiation. Vitamin C is also an antihistamine; by inhibiting histamine release and the resulting inflammation, it decreases tumor promotion. In studies of several tumor lines, a combination of vitamins C and B inhibited tumor growth in 50 percent of the treated subjects.

Related to vitamin C is vitamin P. This vitamin is in the white rind and pulp of citrus fruits and vegetables and amounts to a collection of some 3,000 substances, or family members. What they all have in common is that they make the red and blue colors in plants. Vitamin P increases the absorption of vitamin C; the two should be taken together. You should suspect a deficiency if your pet has blood vessels that break easily, skin that shows many bruises, bleeding gums, or loose teeth; is anemic; or retains fluid. Time-released types are good choices because they maintain a constant higher level of vitamin C in the body. If you're worried about vitamin C supplements and the possibility of kidney stone formation, add a magnesium supplement to the mix. An inefficient form of vitamin C comes from products that have too much binder and filler; under these circumstances, the vitamin cannot be absorbed in the digestive tract and then reabsorbed by the kidneys. Antibiotics, aspirin, antihistamines, barbiturates, and synthetic estrogen all act to destroy vitamin C. Even though dogs make vitamin C, I would recommend that city dogs be given supplemental vitamin C daily.

Vitamin C content in food deteriorates rapidly. To minimize loss, buy fresh fruits and vegetables when they are in season, store them in the refrigerator, and use them as soon as possible. Don't let food stand in water. Cook vitamin C–rich vegetables in a minimal amount of water and never in copper or iron cookware. In short, vitamin C minimizes DNA damage and oxidative stress.

VITAMIN E

The scores of books written about vitamin E testify to its importance as an antioxidant. So vital is it that other vitamins and nutrients will sacrifice themselves to keep up vitamin E levels in the body. This vitamin makes up a family of eight naturally occurring compounds with Greek names called tocopherols, plus a number of minor players called tocotrienols. It is a fat-soluble vitamin that acts more like a water-soluble one. Vitamin E is related to another powerful chemical family called the polyphenols. Within this family are found the antioxidant catechins—green tea extract being one example—and proanthocyanidins, such as grape seed extract. And, interestingly, it is related to the citrus bioflavonoids. Vitamin E, coupled with the mineral selenium, is the first line of defense against free radical damage.

One big role that vitamin E plays relates to the aging process. Studies show that high levels of supplementary vitamin E reverse the decline in immunological responsiveness that occurs with aging. Because vitamins A and C are very sensitive to the presence of oxygen, they can lose much of their value over time. But the presence of E protects them from overoxidation. Vitamin E appears to protect against muscle degeneration, anemia, and the destruction of red blood cells and against certain chronic diseases, such as coronary heart disease.

Naturally occurring vitamin E is usually prefixed with a "d-" as in "d-alpha tocopherol," while the synthetic version is usually preceded by "dl-." Your dog is likely to respond better to a natural E supplement because more of it is bioavailable, it is retained longer in the body tissues, and it is more potent overall.

Chemicals used in treating water (e.g., chlorine), as well as antibiotics, iron supplements, and high levels of fat in the diet, reduce the levels of vitamin E. Start using this vitamin if your pet's levels are low, particularly if he has been diagnosed with hyperthyroidism, diabetes, heart disease, or high blood pressure. High doses of the vitamin can decrease platelet aggregation or clumping and, when given with NSAIDs, can act to thin the blood.

In short, vitamin E reduces oxidative stress.

THE B VITAMINS

The B vitamin family is composed of 11 different nutrients. This is why you'll hear vitamin B referred to as a complex. All the B vitamins are important. They work synergistically and are more potent together than when used singly. Giving too much of one family member can result in a deficiency of the others. In any condition or situation where your pet is under stress (an illness, surgery, trauma, and so on), the need for B vitamins increases dramatically. A little rice polish sprinkled on his food can rapidly replenish missing B vitamins.

This family of nutrients affects a broad variety of body systems, including the brain, nervous system, blood cells, muscles, skin, hair and fur, and the endocrine system. Activities it affects include glucose conversion, protection against radiation exposure, repair of tissue damage, stimulation of cell growth, production of myelin insulation of the nerves, and the metabolization of amino acids, minerals, fats, and proteins. It is also a coenzyme in many body processes.

This vitamin is destroyed by many commonly used drugs: steroids, antiseizure medication, hormone replacement therapy medication, antibiotics, sulfonamides, antidiabetic medication, and NSAIDs. Because they are water soluble, they are not stored and must be replenished daily. In short, vitamin B minimizes DNA damage.

HOW TO SUPPLEMENT

In general, no matter what vitamins you give your pet, be sure to store them properly.

Always keep them someplace dry, with a temperature range between 59°F and 86°F.

Because some are light sensitive, protect them, when kept for long-term use, from exposure to light. Don't store them in the refrigerator if giving them on a daily basis: moisture can build up in the bottle and settle on tablets as the bottle is removed, opened, and then stored again in the cold. However, it's fine to keep vitamins in the refrigerator when you're not using them every day. When you do resume daily supplementing, just let the bottle stand at room temperature for a while before opening. To guard against moisture spoilage, place a few kernels of uncooked rice in the bottle. Once opened, vitamins can be used for up to 12 months. Unopened, the shelf life is two to three years.

Taking the right vitamins at the right time is much more important than previously realized. If your pet is aging, has fallen ill or is recovering from an illness, or has a chronic disease, it is a good time to start adding vitamins to his life. Moreover, we can easily go beyond this thinking to the next logical step: using vitamins as deterrents to aging, deterioration, and disease initiation. The conditions of our lives today have made the use of vitamins almost mandatory. We can keep our pets healthier, stronger, and happier at all times if we provide their cells with the right tools.

Ever since the first vitamin, vitamin A, was chemically isolated in 1913, our knowledge of how important these micronutrients are has expanded dramatically. Initially, it was merely recognized that vitamins helped prevent diseases, such as beriberi and scurvy, when adequately represented in the diet. Research has added much more to our understanding of how big a role they play in preventing killer diseases. Researchers at the M.D. Anderson Hospital and Tumor Institute in Texas report that the use of various nutrients, particularly a B complex with extra B1, B2, B3, folic acid, and vitamin K, helped prevent malnutrition, a common consequence of conventional cancer care and a major cause of death. Lung cancer patients given large doses of vitamin A, beta-carotene, vitamin E, vitamin D, the whole family of B vitamins, vitamin C, fatty acids and minerals—23 nutrients in all—were still alive at the end of the three-year study and had tolerated chemotherapy well. It appears that the earlier cancer patients start taking nutritional supplements, the more likely they are to survive.

Vitamins do not replace food; rather, they need food in order to be assimilated. Once in the mouth, food goes through a process of continuous chemical simplification; as it passes through the digestive tract, it is broken down into smaller and simpler chemical fragments. Macronutrients become micronutrients. The balance between the macro- and microcomponents equals the level of health and proper functioning of the whole system.

Each vitamin has very distinct benefits; thus, there's a lot more to planning a good vitamin regimen than just picking a bottle of multivitamins off the store shelf. Vitamins received their alphabet-based designation because, when first discovered, their chemical structure was undetermined, so they couldn't be given a scientific name. Those that are currently known form family groups; we are only now beginning to understand that there is no one vitamin A, B, or C. That's why we now refer to them as complexes.

The entire spectrum includes the following:

- *A:* A complex referred to as retinols, plus precursors called carotenes
- *B complex:* 11 members, including vitamin G, or vitamin B2; vitamin H, or biotin; and vitamin M, or folic acid
- *C and P:* The P (for "permeability") forms are the bioflavonoids
- *E complex*
- *F:* Fatty acids family

- *K:* Menadione
- *T:* Growth-promoting substances
- *U:* Extracted from cabbage juice

Since most vitamins are the water-soluble type, they can't be stored in the body. A major step in modern vitamin manufacturing was the introduction of time-released supplements. Without time release, the water-soluble types are in and out of the bloodstream within two to four hours. Fat-soluble vitamins remain in the body for almost 24 hours. The optimum time to give vitamins is related to when your pet eats: water soluble between or after meals and fat soluble before them. Since they are organic in nature, vitamins should be taken with other organic substances.

Be sure to read the label because what you are getting along with a vitamin will either help or hinder bioavailability. Fillers or diluents are added to increase bulk. If the filler is dicalcium phosphate, which itself is a source of the mineral calcium, then you receive an added benefit. Binders hold the powdered material of the vitamin together. Usually, cellulose, a plant fiber; gum arabic, a vegetable gum; or seaweed derivatives are used.

Some disagree with the contention that food-based or food-compound vitamins are better than synthetic ones. Let's take a detailed look at the evidence, beginning with the basics.

Vitamins are organic substances and must be included in the diet because they are not made in the body. (An exception is vitamin C, which is made in the canine species.) Vitamins are never isolated in nature; that is, in their natural form, they are food complexes and come primarily from plant tissue.

On the opposite side of the vitamin question is the United States Pharmacopeia (USP) synthetic vitamins. They are isolates, made in the laboratory, usually in the form of crystals. They don't originate from plants. USP vitamins are not food, they have little and sometimes no interaction with each other or with ingested food, and they are manufactured by the same companies that make medicinal drugs.

Whenever we take or give our pets vitamins, minerals, or trace elements, we want to know if these nutrients will be used by the body to perform their necessary work. Because vitamins and other nutrients are subjected to a great number of influences in the course of processing, harvesting, and such—events that affect their bioavailability or usage—we need to know which kind—the synthetic, the natural, or the food based—will work at or near 100 percent capacity.

One influencing factor in utilization is size: the smaller the particle size, the better its absorption. USP vitamins have more nonabsorbable components than food-based vitamins do. Moreover, USP vitamins are not chemically related to natural vitamins. They are synthesized and standardized and haven't been proven to safely replace all natural vitamin activities. As to safety, some currently utilized synthetic vitamins are suspected of having the potential to cause problems. There is evidence that some USP vitamins have left users with symptoms of deficiency, some have been shown to produce no vitamin activity at all, and some even act as antagonists to the absorption of other vitamins.

Looking at the most familiar vitamins, we find some eye-opening information:

Vitamin A

- Vitamin A exists in food in the form of esters (fats) and synthetically as an acid.
- Vitamin A makes up a large number of metabolites called retinols as well as a large number of clones with structural similarities; the synthetic version comes as a single, isolated chemical called retinoic acid.
- Some synthetic versions are suspected of having the potential to cause cirrhosis and, in doses of more than 10,000 international units (IUs) per day, increased the rate of birth defects. Consumption of over 10,000 IUs per day of natural vitamin A in the form of beta-carotene did not.
- The major synthetic form of vitamin A is a vinyl or part coal-tar derivative at some state in its processing, depending on the manufacturer.
- Studies on synthetic vitamin A concluded that this form significantly reduced the level of vitamin E in the body; food-based forms enhanced and helped recycle vitamin E.
- USP vitamin A is more toxic than natural-food-complex vitamin A.
- Food-based vitamin A is one and a half times more absorbable than the synthetic version.

The Vitamin B Family

- Vitamin B1 is a base in its food-based form. When synthesized, it becomes a solid salt that has been processed with ammonia and, at some point in the process, was a coal-tar derivative.

- Studies have found that natural-food-complex vitamin B1 is absorbed 1.38 times better and retained 1.27 times better than the isolated synthetic form.
- The free form of vitamin B2 is a base; in the synthetic form, it becomes a solid with very little vitamin activity.
- The food-complex form was absorbed and retained almost two times more than the isolated form.
- Vitamin B3, or niacinamide, in natural form doesn't cause the gastrointestinal upset or liver toxicity that time-released synthetic niacin can.
- Synthetic vitamin B3 is usually made by a process involving the use of formaldehyde and ammonia.
- Natural-food-complex niacinamide is almost four times more absorbable and retained than the isolate form.
- Synthetic vitamin B5 involves the use of formaldehyde in its processing.
- At least one synthetic vitamin B6 has been found to inhibit natural vitamin B6 action.
- The synthetic form usually requires formaldehyde in its production.
- Natural-food-complex vitamin B6 is two and a half times more absorbable than the isolate form.
- Use of synthetic folic acid, or vitamin B9, may put people and pets at risk for vitamin B12 deficiency. Using more than 200 milligrams of the common USP product called pteroylglutamic acid (PGA) can result in the interference of natural folate metabolism for years.
- Vitamin B12 in the synthetic form has been shown to be antagonistic to naturally occurring vitamin B12.
- Natural-food-based vitamin B12 is absorbed 2.56 times more and retained 1.5 times more than the synthetic version.
- The synthetic form is made through a fermentation process that involves the addition of cyanide.

Vitamin C

- Vitamin C complex in food is absorbed 1.74 times better into red blood cells than isolate USP ascorbic acid.

Vitamin D

- Vitamin D is not an isolate but a combination of forms. Since vitamin D isn't very stable, manufacturers can put in one and a half to two times as much synthetic vitamin D, something that can lead to neonatal problems and hypercalcemia.

Vitamin E

- Food-based vitamin E has roughly twice the availability of synthetic vitamin E.
- Food-based vitamin E is absorbed 3.42 times better than synthetic vitamin E.

The primary reason that isolated USP vitamins were developed was cost; a secondary reason was standardization and stability. It's harder to standardize food. However, neither reason justifies placing isolates on the same nutritional level as vitamins found in food, nor would we want to digest most of the materials used to make and process synthetic vitamins, such as coal tar, ammonia, arsenic, or cyanide. There is even some evidence suggesting that some of these synthetics may be harmful; they are unquestionably less effective. The body can tell whether a vitamin in the bloodstream came from an organically grown apple or from a chemist's laboratory. Given that synthetic vitamins can't match the protective effects of food-based ones, it makes sense to spend your resources on what works.

It's best to get as many as possible of our micronutrients the most natural way—through the food that we eat. Two or three servings daily of "power food"—broccoli, cauliflower, cabbage, Brussels sprouts, mustard greens, turnips, or broccoli rabe—give the body its most valuable allies in the form of antioxidant, anti-inflammatory, antiallergy, antiviral, and anti-cancer agents. Variety is the key; each fruit and vegetable brings its own set of chemicals to the table. Variety offers protection against deficiencies in any of the nutrients we need. Studies show and support the theory of a reduced risk for site-specific cancers in relation to the intake of select vegetables and fruit.[4] Some examples follow:

Colorectal cancer: Cruciferous vegetables and vegetables and fruit rich in folate (B vitamin)
Gastric/stomach: Green-yellow vegetables
Esophageal: Vegetables and fruits rich in vitamin C
Lungs: Carotenoid-rich vegetables and fruits

Pancreas: Folate-rich vegetables and fruits
Prostate: Tomato

Has your pet had his kale today?

There are many foods that can be included in pet diets to boost their vitamin levels. The best food sources of vitamin A are the following:

Alfalfa
Beets
Broccoli
Cantaloupe
Carrots
Dandelion greens
Kale
Parsley
Pumpkin
Spinach
Sweet potato

The best food sources of B vitamins are the following:

Alfalfa
Brown rice
Brussels sprouts
Lentils
Lima beans
Oats
Peas (fresh)
Seeds
Soy
Wheat germ

The best food sources of vitamin C are the following:

Beet greens
Broccoli
Cantaloupe

Green peas
Kale
Parsley
Spinach
Tomatoes
Turnip
Watercress

The best food sources of vitamin E are the following:

Brown rice
Cornmeal
Dry beans
Eggs
Leafy green vegetables
Nuts
Oatmeal
Wheat germ

The best food sources of carotenes are the following:

Apricots
Broccoli
Cantaloupe
Carrots
Collard greens
Kale
Parsley
Spinach
Sweet potato
Tomatoes
Watermelon

The best food sources of flavonoids are the following:

Apples (with the skin)
Blueberries

Broccoli
Cranberries
Parsley
Raspberries
Strawberries
Zucchini

The best food sources of the five major carotenoids are the following:

- *Alpha-carotene:* Pumpkin and carrots
- *Beta-carotene:* Sweet potatoes, carrots, apricots, spinach, collard greens, pumpkin, and cantaloupe
- *Beta-cryptoxanthin*: Papaya, oranges, and tangerines
- *Lutein and zeaxanthin:* Kale, collard greens, spinach, Swiss chard, mustard greens, red peppers, okra, and romaine lettuce
- *Lycopene:* Tomatoes, watermelon, guava, and pink grapefruit

GREENS

Adding greens to your pet's diet provides him with additional nutrients. It's easy to grow greens at home. In the late spring and through summer and fall, you can buy greens, but it becomes harder to get young, organic greens in the winter. This is the time to think of an indoor garden.

You can start with small pots on a windowsill in your kitchen. Plant a few seeds of each vegetable in every pot. As the early leaves emerge throughout the winter, you can feed them to your dog, cat, or bird. Start the process with good-quality soil; organic is best. Purchase seed packets that have been left over the summer; these are usually less expensive but still have good growth potential.

Plantings can be chosen for their dark green color, but if you have introduced your pet to greens during the summer, you will have an idea of which plants he may favor. Some pets show preferences for collards, mustard greens, beet greens, turnip greens, or spinach. You can harvest leaves for cooking and mixing into the meal each day. For birds, you can add large leaves through the cage bars both for the entertainment he may get from tearing the leaves apart and for nourishment.

MINERALS

Vitamins are not the only natural agents our bodies require to maintain optimal health and fight disease. The minerals selenium and zinc, while important in a wide variety of biological processes, are particularly significant with respect to cancer. Selenium has been pointed out to be particularly important since numerous studies suggest that an inverse association exists between selenium levels and the incidence of cancer. Humans and animals with the lowest selenium levels are twice as likely to develop cancer as those with the highest levels. Selenium deficiency is very much linked to geography. Humans and animals living in areas where soil and crops contain high levels of selenium are less likely to get head and neck, lung, colon, or breast cancer. In a five-year study in an area of China with a high incidence of primary liver cancer, selenium supplementation significantly reduced this rate.[5] In women over age 50, selenium supplementation provides a preventive effect against breast cancer.[6] The answer to why selenium works may be found in the fact that deficiency levels open the body to low immune system effectiveness. Selenium protects against the toxic effects of most heavy metals: cadmium, mercury, lead, and arsenic. In concert with zinc, it helps conserve and recycle vitamin E. The primary enzyme that converts hydrogen peroxide to water and prevents fat peroxidation is selenium dependent.

Zinc is required by more than 100 enzymes as well as for the proper functioning of T-lymphocytes. Zinc deficiency leads to atrophy of the thymus gland and decreased activity of the NK cells. Zinc and immunity are intimately linked. Scientists from Michigan State University found that without enough zinc, the body may lose its ability to remember what it has been immunized against. A special part of the immune system, the memory cells, may be destroyed when zinc is deficient, making successful vaccinations against common diseases impossible.

Iron is important to a pet's ability to ward off infections. Phagocytes, white blood cells that serve as the first line of defense in a bacterial infection, depend on iron-containing enzymes to work. Phagocytes need plenty of oxygen in order to engulf bacteria and secrete a variety of corrosive substances that will digest the invading microbe. Iron provides the fuel.

Lymphocytes, another white blood cell group, need iron to play their specialized role in the immune response. Iron is also important to brain function. Motivation to persist in intellectually challenging tasks may be lowered, attention span shortened, and overall intellectual performance diminished in an iron-deficient body.

Absorption is critical for providing enough iron. There are two kinds: heme and nonheme. Heme iron is the easiest to absorb and comes primarily from meat, fish, and liver. An anemic animal can be fed liver if the food source is organically raised meat or chicken. Nonheme-type iron are iron compounds found in vegetables and grains. Adding about 60 milligrams of vitamin C to a meal of rice will more than triple iron absorption. Vitamin C can come from food additions, such as tomatoes; broccoli; leafy green vegetables, such as kale; turnip tops; and collard greens, as well as seasonings, such as lemon juice or parsley. Adding papaya enzymes to a meal will boost iron absorption by 500 percent.

Sulfur plays by far one of the biggest roles in detoxifying your or your pet's body. Usually, this mineral doesn't need to be supplemented if the diet has enough protein; its derivatives, including certain amino acids or collagen-building substances, such as glucosamine sulfate, are everywhere. When it comes to chemical compounds, it would be difficult to find one that is older or that has a more colorful history than sulfur. Biochemists believe that sulfur played a role in the first creation of life on land by making possible photosynthesis, a way that very primitive life forms could breathe air. Later, sulfur reinvented itself into a very different essential part of living systems. Some three or more billion years ago, it took on a number of additional forms. Whenever you see "thio" in a nutrient's name, you know it is a sulfur compound. For example, metallothionein is a sulfur compound that stores and regulates zinc, which in turn binds itself to heavy metals, such as mercury, and rids the body of this toxic metal. In fact, all sulfur derivatives act as scavengers.

Long-term, low-level exposure to toxins leads to disease. As far back as 1979, the Environmental Protection Agency published warnings that we face real danger from our constant exposure to harmful elements. You can find out how affected you or your pet are via hair analysis. This test is available for humans and dogs; it looks at trace mineral levels in the body and gives an excellent picture of the state of toxicity. Blood and urine analyses do not. Hair or fur (the latter in the case of most dogs) locks metals into its structure. A fur sample analysis will assess the overall status of body nutrients as well as toxin levels. You are then well positioned to begin the process of detoxification and/or nutrient supplementation.

8

MORE ON ANTIOXIDANTS
AND CANCER

A central focus of any cancer-fighting program has to be the patient's internal biochemistry. One's body can either nourish cancer cells or send them to their death. Targeting a tumor surgically may be all a patient needs of conventional medicine, but if malignant cells are left behind, the cancer can then begin again. Your pet's internal chemical environment plays an integral part in determining whether a tumor will regain its foothold after treatment, stay dormant, or even be killed.

The internal environment surrounding precancerous and cancerous cells influences the outcome by being hospitable or inhospitable to growth. What environmental factors matter? And what can be done to establish the healthiest terrain possible?

Issues to be addressed are inflammation, free radical buildup, nutritional deficiencies, and immunity. If you know of or suspect problems in the state of your pet's internal environment, you'll want to learn how you can change his biochemistry to create an environment hostile to cancer's growth and spread.

Let's look at some easy-to-use natural agents that are proven anticancer effective and cancer preventive as well. The bioflavonoid silymarin, a constituent of the herb milk thistle, is one. In a retrospective study of 405 human patients with metastatic brain lesions, supplements with fish oil (3 grams a day) and silymarin (200 milligrams per day) resulted in a

64 percent increase in survival duration compared to unsupplemented patients.[1] Boswellia, an Ayurvedic herb, can be taken as an adjunct to treatment in brain tumors. This agent markedly inhibits tumor growth in animal studies and increases survival time. Bromelain, from the pineapple, has anti-inflammatory properties and interferes with the growth of malignant cells. This agent's anti-inflammatory effect is comparable to that of the steroid prednisone. Curcumin, or turmeric, has a long history of use in the treatment of inflammatory disorders. Curcumin appears to exhibit antiproliferative effects in a variety of human cancer cell lines, including hormone-dependent cancers. Curcumin influences and induces apoptosis (cell death). In animal studies, curcumin increases the life span of rodents with transplanted tumors, inhibiting tumor growth and impeding metastasis. It has been shown to enhance natural killer (NK) cell mediation. Quercetin, a plant flavonol, is the major bioflavonoid in our diet. Its documented activities include inhibition of tumor growth and increased life span in tumor-bearing animals. Quercetin has demonstrated significant antitumor activity against a wide range of cancers, including brain tumors, lung cancers, and stomach and colon cancers.[2]

Giving your pet a combination that includes as many of these agents as possible every day is the first step toward making his internal biochemistry as hostile as possible to cancer cells. A combination formula that includes the needed agents can minimize pill giving. Then, depending on the situation, build on this foundation with specific terrain boosters and modifiers targeting one or more particular aspects of the terrain.

OXIDATION

As I mentioned earlier, back in 1954, Dr. Denham Harmon recognized that free radical reactions were an inevitable part of the oxidation process: as long as life requires oxygen, there is "rusting," or oxidation, that takes place. Harmon theorized that reducing free radical damage would require two things: either a decrease in the rate at which oxidation takes place or an interruption in the process. Decreasing the rate of oxidation appears to be connected to food intake: restrict food intake and don't serve your pet certain foods, such as fats and sugars. Interruption is accomplished through antioxidants. These agents sacrifice themselves, giving up their electron to the free radical molecule and, in the process, aborting cellular damage.

The protective role of antioxidant activity is critical to health in general but even more crucial to cells, such as those of the brain, retina, and arteries. These cells are impossible to replace.

The body does make antioxidants, but the majority of these need to be supplemented to make up for the results of poor diet, stress, nutritional deficiencies, chronic disease, therapeutic drugs, and other factors. Some antioxidants come from vitamins, and some come from minerals, amino acids, and plant or natural botanical substances.

Cancer cells produce free radicals at a higher-than-normal rate. Free radicals break strands of DNA and mix up chromosomes during cell division. They damage the endothelial cells that line blood vessels, making it easier for tumor cells to enter this highway to metastasis. They help tumors grow the blood vessels they need and are partially responsible for changing the cells' internal communication network, fostering out-of-control proliferation. The proliferation of free radicals, which is a side effect of chemotherapy and radiation and evidence of a drug's resistance to chemotherapy agents, may lead to a likelihood that cancer will reappear as secondary tumors.[3] Ralph Moss, PhD, formerly of the Sloan-Kettering Cancer Treatment Center, states the criteria for measuring the effectiveness of a given cancer treatment. "If it only temporarily shrinks tumors, with a probable loss in well-being, then it is at most entirely experimental and unproven and should not be represented as anything else. At worse, it could be not just ineffective, but painful, destructive—even fatal."

Don't depend on an oncologist to explain and help you sort out what you need for free radical protection. Indeed, many oncologists believe that the use of antioxidants along with conventional care will counteract the effectiveness of chemotherapy. Chemotherapy and radiation therapy produce high amounts of free radicals; patients taking antioxidants in tandem do better. Neither survival nor tumor shrinkage has been shown to be significantly worse with antioxidant use. In fact, studies strongly suggest that antioxidants make it easier for patients to tolerate all their necessary rounds of chemotherapy without having to stop because of adverse side effects.

The free radical proliferation generated by chemotherapy and radiation attacks healthy tissues, too. When chemotherapy drugs attack nerve cells, damage called neuropathy can result. This condition usually affects the extremities, resulting in tingling, numbness, and even pain. Chemo-induced free radicals can damage heart muscle. Inflammation of the rectum that results in diarrhea, rectal pain, rectal bleeding, and even fecal incontinence can be induced by radiation. To minimize free radical damage to normal tissues, we need to employ multiple strategies.

The only way you can change your pet's internal environment is through biochemical agents. The conventional medical world doesn't have a pill for this. But you have many options, thanks to alternative medicine.

If possible, you can make a case with your pet's oncologist to compose a program of low-dose chemotherapy—very small doses spread out over a longer period of time—and to treat your pet with herbal therapy. Survival rates improve significantly in patients with lung, breast, throat, stomach, and nasopharyngeal cancers when paired with Chinese herbs (95 percent vs. 79 percent).[4]

FLAVONOIDS

Antioxidant activity can be general, or it can be tissue specific. Vitamins, such as C and E, and minerals, such as selenium and zinc, are generally useful antioxidants for the body as a whole. But another group, the flavonoids, are highly effective in healing specific tissues: each individual member concentrates on one particular part, be it the brain, the vascular linings, the lungs, the pancreas, the eyes, the liver, the heart, or elsewhere. Flavonoids are a family of nutrients capable of highly specific biological action. Many members of the family have the ability to concentrate on a particular body system and its problems, while others will combat allergies, viruses, and cancers.

Flavonoids, the active ingredients in many plants, are found mostly in the leaves, flowers, and fruits of these plants. For a long time, they were not considered important from a medical standpoint, but now, as researchers gain a deeper understanding of how they work, their medicinal value is becoming much more widely recognized.

Two subgroups of flavonoids, the catechins and the quercetins, are highly effective in protecting the body's internal terrain. They can inactivate many viruses, including those that cause herpes simplex and numerous respiratory problems. Others protect against molds and gastrointestinal infections, such as thrush and yeast. Still others inhibit the body's allergy mechanism, which is responsible for the itching, runny nose, and sneezing discomfort of allergies. Thus, flavonoids are often used by alternative practitioners to treat asthma and sinus congestion. Certain subgroup members work on the skin, soothing rashes and protecting against the rejection of skin grafts.

The flavonoid family in general is a versatile one. Its members range from the not so familiar, such as rutin and catechin, to the more well known, such as rose hips, citrus peel, and grape seed. One of the best-known flavonoids is gingko biloba.

Gingko biloba is an herb with powerful antioxidant effects in the brain, retina, and cardiovascular system. It is the leaves and seeds of the plant that are used. This herb improves brain functioning by increasing cerebral circulation; I often use it in herbal combinations to treat dogs that have suffered a stroke or show signs of confusion and inattention as they age. This plant also increases blood flow to the limbs and is used in peripheral arterial disease, in which arteries are obstructed and narrowed by plaque. Gingko is safe and can be used long term. In fact, the longer it is used, the more benefit it imparts, particularly as an antioxidant. The cell membranes in your pet's body are the first line of defense in protecting the cell's integrity, erecting fluid barriers to pathogens and free radicals. These membranes are themselves susceptible to damage, but flavonoids, such as gingko, provide protection.

I mentioned previously that research has shown the combination of vitamins C and E to have especially strong value as antioxidants. One category of flavonoids, known as the proanthocyanidins, has an even stronger effect. Within this subgroup, two agents rise head and shoulders above the rest: grape seed extract and the bark of the French maritime pine tree. (Technically, they are oligomeric proanthocyanidins [OPCs]—food or botanical sources of unique phytochemicals having powerful antioxidant capabilities.) This group is highly water soluble and rapidly absorbed and utilized in the body. Some tests suggest that these OPCs may be as much as 50 times more potent than vitamin E and 20 times more potent than vitamin C in terms of bioavailable antioxidant activity.[5] Every member of the group works with glutathione to recycle and restore vitamin C.

Extracts from the seeds of the wine grape protect pets against age-related damage and cancer. Japanese researchers have found significant inhibitory effects on the abnormal growth of cells as well as the suppression of tumor cells. This agent is credited with treating DNA fragmentation and hydrogen peroxide–induced injury to white blood cells and especially brain cells. The OPCs protect the vascular system by trapping free radicals and lipid (fat) peroxides, slowing down the destruction of arteries.

Numerous studies demonstrate that an individual's level of antioxidants may be a more significant factor in determining the risk of developing heart disease than his lipid levels.

Grape seed extract helps to regulate the actions of the genes that control the normal life of individual cells. In the cell, it has two important roles: one is the slowing of aging by keeping free radical levels low, and the other is cytotoxicity, the killing off of abnormal cells.

The other proanthocyanidin is the French maritime pine bark extract patented as Pycnogenol. The extract contains approximately 40 natural ingredients. It is very effective used separately, but when taken in combination with alpha-lipoic acid and vitamins C and E, it becomes one of the most potent antioxidants of all. It also provides most of the benefits of grape seed extract, particularly for the cardiovascular system.

Gingko biloba, red grape seed extract, and French maritime pine bark extract belong to the catechin family, a subgroup called polyphenols. Green tea extract and garlic are also catechin family members. On the whole, all these natural agents are particularly powerful disease fighters and potent antioxidants.

Other important members of the flavonoid group are to be found in the thistle family, milk thistle and artichoke being at the top. Milk thistle is to the liver what calcium is to the bones: absolutely necessary. It will detoxify the liver and stimulate liver cell regeneration. Combine it with glutathione for a cleaning and with vitamin C for cell change. In chronic liver conditions, such as hepatitis, cirrhosis, and cancer, survival rates are higher when the animal's diet is supplemented with milk thistle and artichoke. (It should be noted that the treatment of liver conditions also requires high amounts of dietary fiber with food to expedite the elimination of bile acids and any medicinal drugs that may have been given.)

The thistle family makes up a group of flavonoid compounds; its main component is silymarin. Silymarin extracted from the seeds of the herb has been used for centuries to treat liver disease. Modern research shows that it is effective in treating both acute and chronic viral liver disease. Silymarin guards the liver from oxidative damage and protects it from the toxins in drugs. At the same time, it can promote the growth of new liver cells. As an added benefit, it increases the levels of glutathione in the body. Milk thistle is very low in toxicity and can be given over long periods of time, sometimes even for the rest of the animal's life.

Artichoke extract is in many ways similar to milk thistle; silymarin plus cymarin are active ingredients in both. Providing artichoke extract as a supplement can turn around cases in which an animal's digestion is poor because his liver is not producing enough bile. This herb definitely helps the dyspeptic animal, the severely constipated animal, and the colicky animal. It will stop vomiting, diminish abdominal pain, improve appetite, and reduce gas. It can relieve irritable bowel syndrome and the associated pain, altered bowel functions, and excessive secretion of mucus in the colon.

Every time the liver has to neutralize a toxin, the liver is damaged somewhat in the process. The effective way to protect the liver and eliminate the toxin as quickly as possible is through increasing the volume of bile. This bile will carry the toxins out of the body through the digestive tract. In studies, artichoke extract has been shown to increase the flow of bile by more than 100 percent in minutes, with no incidence of toxicity.

Animals with gallbladder problems, such as stones, gravel, or inflammation, can suffer from digestive disturbances. A diet low in fiber or high in fat is linked to poor bile flow, along with treatment with steroids, estrogen hormone replacement, aspirin, and some antibiotics. Impaired bile flow shows up as general malaise, allergies, constipation, and digestive changes. These symptoms reveal a subclinical stage of poor liver function that doesn't show up in blood tests. Since both milk thistle and artichoke are tonics for the liver, gallbladder, and bile ducts, they are often used interchangeably.

OTHER NATURAL BIOCHEMICAL AGENTS

Alpha lipoic acid, a powerful universal antioxidant that functions in both the membrane and the aqueous part of cells, scavenges and reduces several types of oxidation. In addition, it recycles vitamins C and E, coenzyme Q10 (CoQ10), and glutathione levels. It is naturally found in the body and is both water and fat soluble. Supplemental alpha lipoic acid has been used for almost three decades in Europe to treat peripheral nerve degeneration and to help control blood sugar levels in people with diabetes. It helps detoxify the liver of metal pollutants. And it is very useful in poststroke treatment plans. In a stroke, millions of cells die, resulting in an extraordinary number of free radicals that if left unchecked continue to engage in more and more destruction in the area.

An aging animal can benefit from alpha lipoic acid supplements because the body makes less and less of it as it ages. It is found in only a few food sources, so supplementation is probably necessary. It's too soon to be sure, but this antioxidant may act to inhibit the replication of viruses in the body. If this promise proves true, it may be useful in the treatment of cats with damaging viral conditions.

CoQ10 is exceptionally useful both for its antioxidant value and as a biochemical system modifier. It is found in every cell of the body and is involved in the production of energy. When it is subclinically lacking over a long period of time, the deficiency can be an invitation to heart disease, arterial damage, high blood pressure, and tissue degeneration anywhere in the body. Half of animals with heart disease have drastically low levels of CoQ10, which has become recognized as the treatment of choice for heart disease in many countries.

Soon after CoQ10 was discovered in 1957, it became obvious that this biochemical was essential to the body's production of energy on the most basic level—the cells' mitochondria.

CoQ10 protects the internal integrity of cell membranes. Twenty years of research have shown its protective effects on RNA and DNA repair and enhancement of cellular immunity. CoQ10 inhibits the proliferation of cancer cells into the heart and can protect the heart from damage during conventional cancer treatment.

Hailed as one of the "greats" in antioxidant and anticancer effectiveness, Cellular Forte with IP-6 decreases the number of bad cells by dramatically increasing the activity of NK cells. The main task of NK cells is to hunt down and kill abnormal and virus-infected cells. In clinical trials, Cellular Forte with IP-6 increased NK cells' activity by 50 percent.[6] An alternate approach to cancer is to modify abnormal cell differentiation, or the way these cells grow and mature. This agent doesn't kill cancer cells per se; instead, it slows down the growth of malignant cells so that instead of reproducing wildly and growing profusely, they mature and die just as normal cells do. This decreases bad cellular proliferation; as bad cells mature, this agent causes an eventual reversion of bad cells to the normal type. For example, when the effects of Cellular Forte with IP-6 on fibrosarcoma were studied, researchers found that the tumors of the test subjects got smaller, as many of the cells making up the tumor matured and died off.

Saponins are another general class of plant compounds. Because saponins contain steroids, they can be transformed into cortisone, estrogen, and progesterone when ingested and can be substituted in situations where pharmaceutical steroid hormones might be damaging. Some pharmaceutical steroids, when taken in large doses or for extended periods of time, can damage red blood cells by slipping into the cells and breaking them up. Plant steroids lack these and other side effects of synthetic steroids.

Saponins offer many benefits. They are antioxidants. They can correct the hormonal deficiencies that come with aging. Saponins support the adrenal glands, which handle stress, and boost low gonad steroid levels related to autoimmune disease and the depression of specific white blood cells made in the thymus. (The thymus makes the category of white cells called T-cells, which, in turn, produce the helper cells and the suppressor T-cells. The ratio of helper T-cells to suppressor T-cells indicates the status of the immune system. If the ratio is low, immunodeficiency is present. If the ratio is high, an autoimmune disease may be present.) The best-known sources of saponins are soybeans and peas.

As a group, "green" foods include wheatgrass and barley grass, oats, cereal grasses, and sea microalgae—all characterized by their pigment. Because of their unique chlorophyll pigment structure, green foods supply a high amount of nutrients. Their chlorophyll structure is almost identical to the structure of hemoglobin, a vital component in blood. Introducing greens into a diet fuels the blood's delivery of more oxygen to the body. In a study dating back to 1936, animals fed chlorophyll-rich foods combined with iron regenerated red blood cells quickly, making greens a possible treatment for deficiency anemia.

Green foods contain all the amino acids; they alkalize cells, and they work with probiotics to improve the body's absorption of nutrients. They even inhibit the growth of harmful bacteria.

Sea algae, such as blue-green algae, spirulina, and chlorella, stimulate the production of NK cells in your pet's immune system. These cells go after and destroy virus-infected cells, especially in the spleen, lungs, liver, and gut linings. A substance called astaxanthin, extracted from algae, boosts the immune system and protects cell membranes.

Research suggests that algae stimulate high antioxidant activity and are thought to be able to repair damaged DNA. Extracts of cereal grasses have shown the ability to detoxify cells and eliminate those damaged by carcinogens, chemicals, and toxins. Sweet wheatgrass extract applied to chemicals that are known to cause cancer reduced the chemicals' effect by up to 99 percent. Research on barley grass extract has identified its ability to detoxify pesticides and herbicides.

The common sea algae—spirulina, chlorella, and aphanizomenon flos-aquae—differ only by where they grow in the world. Spirulina is grown in man-made ponds, chlorella is imported from Japan, and aphanizomenon flos-aquae is harvested from natural lakes, such as those in Oregon.

STANDARDS

Once you start looking into antioxidants, you will come to realize that they are specialists, not generalists. That is, you need to combine a number of them to offer the best defense. Since many antioxidants reinforce and/or recycle one another, choosing a complex will supply full-spectrum protection. A rating system devised by the U.S. Department of Agriculture called "Oxygen Radical Absorbency Capacity" can help you put together your pet's individual plan. The higher the number in the rating, the more powerful the antioxidant value of the nutrient. The ratings are based on 3.5-ounce servings. Not surprisingly, broccoli carries a rating of 890, Brussels sprouts 980, spinach 1,260, and kale 1,770. In the fruit aisle, blueberries are rated at 2,400, and prunes at 5,770.

Free radicals and their nemeses, the antioxidants, are cutting-edge science. The number of cells destroyed over the years by free radicals is enormous. Free radicals can literally destroy major organs. By way of illustration, your liver at age 70 will be just half the size it was when you were 25, thanks to the destruction of tissue by free radicals over the course of those intervening years. You need to arm yourself intelligently.

As the preceding has made clear, everything that goes in the mouth has the potential to alter the biochemistry of the body. The processes affected are those that regulate the body; therefore, these substances are called biological response modifiers (BRMs). Food is the best source of BRMs, but, as the nutritional value of our food continues to diminish because of modern farming techniques and overprocessing, the BRM value has declined. To fill the vacuum of missing nutrients, more and more people are turning to supplements. Indeed, there is a plethora of vitamins, minerals, and other nutrients now available in the marketplace. We no longer ask, do we supplement but, rather, what do we supplement with, what are our goals, and what are the proper dosages?

Another factor of equal importance is whether the particular product contains what its label says it does. Independent studies have analyzed various supplements only to find that an alarmingly large number contained little to none of the active ingredient needed for effectiveness. One independent study tested major brands of the popular supplement Saint-John's-wort, an herbal nutritional supplement used for treating mild depression, and found that three brands had no more than half the active ingredient shown on the label. Only four major brands had 90 percent of the active ingredient shown on the label, and only those brands with the highest amount had enough of the herb's components to be effective. Similar tests on other supplements have concluded that some brands were falsely labeled and potentially useless.

However, let me quickly add that the industry as a whole tends to be ethical; many manufacturers and distributors offer excellent products and quality assurance programs, and the industry as a whole has been working with the federal government to put safeguards in place to ensure both safety and quality.

Knowing the amount of the active ingredient in a product is important, as it helps to determine dosage, cost, and effect. Standardization for each individual active ingredient in a phytochemical comes from research. Some of the more popular supplements have their active ingredients well defined:

- Bilberry, for vision health, is 25 percent antocyanosides.
- Grape seed extract, for free radical scavenging, is 95 percent proanthocyanidins.
- Hawthorn berry, for cardiovascular health, is 19 percent OPCs.
- Gingko biloba, for brain health, is 24 percent flavone glycosides.
- Milk thistle, for liver health, is 70 percent silymarin.

Important information like this should be on the label. However, there is much more to learn about a particular supplement than the active ingredient and its standardization. A plant contains many compounds, often leading researchers to believe that the whole is greater than its parts. It could matter a great deal if using the whole herb or plant could result in greater benefit than standardizing only one of its active ingredients.

On the label of any of these products, look for the USP symbol; it stands for the United States Pharmacopeia Convention, an organization that analyzes, tests, and monitors supplements. A bottle that shows the USP symbol comes from a manufacturer that complies with the current highest standards. In addition, the label will tell you more:

- Serving size, which could be one or more tablets.
- Amount per serving, for example, alpha lipoic acid at 200 milligrams.
- Percentage of daily value. In this case, there are many supplements that don't have an established daily value; if there is one, it will be listed as a percentage of the Recommended Daily Allowance (RDA) or Reference Daily Intake (RDI).
- Directions for use.
- Listing of other ingredients both active and as binders, fillers, and so on.
- Manufacturer's code or lot number for reference if you have questions about the product.
- Expiration date.
- Storage instructions.
- Information on how to reach the manufacturer or distributor: address, telephone number, fax number, and/or website and e-mail address.
- Secondary information regarding such concerns as animal testing and kosher or vegetarian standards.

When using most supplements on pets, I suggest you start below half the human dose: if the dose is two tablets per day for a human, then you can safely give about a quarter of a tablet for a small dog or cat and half a tablet for a large dog. Watch your pet's reaction, if any, for about four to five days, and if there is none, you can increase the dose: one-half a tablet for a small dog or cat and one tablet for a large dog. Usually, pets can go up to a child's dose, which is usually one-half a human dose.

One piece of information often included is the RDA; however, RDAs are not the answer for chronic issues or cancer. RDAs were the answer to deficiency syndromes in the past but are now out of touch with the reality of widespread subclinical deficiencies and chronic disease. We need to move beyond the simplicity of RDAs to the next generation of nutrition. We want our nutritional supplements to generate optimal health and longevity.

Moreover, minimal standards are of no use if a body system has been damaged. For a hypothetical case that illustrates this, what would happen if one organ system were damaged at the rate of 10 percent per year but repaired itself at the rate of only 9 percent per year? It would function at a lower level with each succeeding year. If there were any further damage to the same system, the rate of repair would fall even lower; with every subsequent hit to the organ, the slide would be ever further downward until the organ system failed and the body was unable to provide needed repairs. What if we were able to change that ratio? If our life-extension strategies could slow the damage rate by 1 percent and speed the repair rate by 1 percent, the damage rate would become 9 percent and the repair rate 10 percent. Repairs would then be keeping up with the damage. This kind of damage minimizing, carried out over the lifetime of your pet, would maintain a manageable balance.

There are general guidelines for supplements. Not all supplements are the same; the best ones contain enough pure, active ingredient to accomplish their missions and have the right delivery systems to get those ingredients where they are needed. As a general rule, even a healthy pet should be given a multivitamin/mineral supplement with alpha lipoic acid, green food mixture, and probiotics (more on the latter soon).

One of the ways in which a qualified practitioner can help you and your pet is by recommending not only an appropriate course of supplements but also a particular brand. You may go shopping for supplements and find several bottles of a popular herb or other supplement at very different prices, but you mustn't assume that they're all of the same quality. When it comes to supplements, accuracy and truth in labeling has not been as closely monitored in the United States as it has been in Europe and, even more disturbing, neither has lack of contamination. Although this concern is in the process of being addressed, it is important to know the manufacturing and distributing sources.

Given the vast number of choices on the market, how do you identify a good brand? The top professionally used products are not available to laypeople. However, if you decide to purchase a product on your own, over the counter, be sure to read the label. Labels may not have all the information you need to make the best choice, but at least you can rule out any brands that contain allergenic food items, such as yeast, corn, wheat, or dairy—unless that ingredient is a necessary part of the formulation, as it is with probiotics. If the label doesn't state that the product is free of artificial colors, preservatives, sugars, and flavors, put it back on the shelf.

Flavonoid Classes	Class Members	Plant Sources
Flavonols	Catechins	Green tea, grape seeds, pine bark
Flavones	Quercetin	Apples, green tea, gingko leaves, grape skins, milk thistle
Proanthocyanidins	Oligomeric catechins	Pine bark, grape seeds, bilberry, gingko
Flavanones	Hesperidin	Citrus peels
Anthocyanins	Cyanidin	Red and black grapes, red wine, bilberries
Flavonolignans	Silymarin	Milk thistle, artichoke
Isoflavones	Genistein, daidzein	Soybeans

9

WHAT ACUPUNCTURE AND HOMEOPATHY CAN DO

There are two medicines to consider when your pet is about to start a cancer program based on Western medicine: acupuncture and homeopathy. In choosing the route of acupuncture, the owner is including in his or her pet's life the world's oldest medicine. There's evidence of its use as far back as 5300 BC. It appears that a mummy (named the "Tyrolean Iceman") was found in the Alps with tattoos over acupuncture points in a sequential prescription used even now for arthritic pain of the back and legs. It's amazing to think of where this person may have been and who worked on him. Equally amazing is the fact that acupuncture has been a continuous, effective system of medicine through centuries. It is particularly relevant to issues that come up with Western medicine cancer treatment.

Acupuncture involves inserting very fine, disposable, solid, stainless-steel needles into the body along clearly expressed routes called meridians. One theory explains the inserted needle as going down to a tiny well containing multiple biochemicals and touching off discrete reactions. Treatment is usually a series of sessions each building on the previous ones; the value is cumulative, with the patient experiencing positive change over time. As an adjunctive medicine to chemotherapy or radiation, acupuncture needs to be on a continuous basis, sometimes twice a week at the beginning to once a week and an eventual tapering off. If you decide to employ acupuncture

in the area of prevention (posttreatment), needling sessions should be programmed every few weeks of the remaining years of your pet's life.

Animals don't mind being needled and will often experience feelings of
sleepiness and a general mellowness. On the whole, they respond more
quickly than humans. The entire process is side effect free.

Acupuncture and homeopathy also are what modern medicine calls
"energy medicine"; that is, the body's energy is manipulated either through
needling or by the use of homeopathy using extremely diluted and highly
potentized remedies. Both systems perceive the body as an energy field,
called "qi" in acupuncture and "vital force" in homeopathy. When a body
is well, energy flows unobstructed everywhere, and one's basic life force is
strong. Depleted or blocked energy is equated with illness; a weak or suppressed vital force is unable to fend off an illness.

Human cancer patients have been using these energy medicines in
integrated plans to maximize overall health for over 50 years. Hundreds
of clinical trials with acupuncture have shown it to be a very effective tool
for the treatment of pain, loss of appetite, nausea, peripheral cytopenia,
weight loss, and diarrhea.[1] Bentley is an example of what can be done
for a cat.

Bentley was brought in with reports from a biopsy and blood work. They
read, "Malignant lymphoma in the liver . . . severe lymphatic portal duct
hepatitis . . . interpretation is that the lesion is malignant rather than an ex-
pression of an inflammatory disorder." Bentley's liver profile showed three
key markers pathologically high: alkaline phosphatase, which is elevated in
diseases of the liver, such as hepatitis and cirrhosis; bilirubin, an indicator
of hidden or occult liver disease; and aspartate phosphatase, which shows
impaired cell membranes. The current readings were as follows:

AST 275; normal range is 17 to 43
ALT 1,075; normal range is 32 to 82
ALK Phos 268; normal range is 15 to 50

Bentley's doctor gave the family the bad news and a prognosis of a matter
of weeks.

At this point, Bentley became my patient. He needed aggressive care
and as much positive intervention as he could tolerate. We began with
weekly acupuncture sessions, daily doses of a Chinese herbal formula that
incorporated milk thistle seed, and a homeopathy remedy once a day to

support him. Turning a sick liver around typically takes months, so I cautioned his owners to anticipate very little for a while. After four months of work, Bentley went through updated blood work. Now his readings showed the following:

AST 174
ALT 668
ALK Phos 199
Bilirubin 0.7; normal range is 0.1 to 1.5

Bentley showed several hopeful signs as well: his appetite came back, he gained weight, and the jaundice disappeared. We reduced his acupuncture treatments from weekly to once every three or four weeks; he continued with his Chinese medical herbs. Approximately one year after his cancer diagnosis, Bentley was no longer showing signs of ill health, and his lab readings kept going down. He outlived the dire prognosis by two years.

In designing a treatment plan, a practitioner needs to discover the energy imbalances in the body, determine where and how far they extend, and identify the causes of the imbalances. It's a whole-body investigation. Cancer often presents with the problem of a weak or suppressed immune system; studies have explored the role of acupuncture in supporting immune functions by increasing blood cell counts and enhancing natural killer (NK) cell activity and leukocyte activity in general.

In 1997, a panel of health experts at the U.S. National Institutes of Health concluded that research results showed acupuncture's efficacy: "There is clear evidence that . . . acupuncture may be effective as an adjunct therapy, an acceptable alternative, or as part of a comprehensive treatment program."[2]

The homeopathic approach pays less attention to the label of the disease than to what the symptom picture is, how the patient experiences the symptoms, what led up to the problem, and the question of who the patient is and how much has his vital energy been impacted. Sandy, a German shepherd, has sarcoma and has been my patient for months. She has been on a homeopathic remedy, hecla lava, throughout, and the tumor has neither grown nor shrunk. The cancer is being managed as a chronic illness. Sandy has been a very healthy animal all her life, and her innate constitution is strong. Her vital force may be able to work with the tumor indefinitely.

Homeopathy began as a medical system with the work of Dr. Samuel Hahnemann in the eighteenth century. He built his medicine on several theories: 1) "like" cures "like" (the "law of similars"), in which a remedy in a minute dose is chosen to treat the symptoms that if taken in a conventional dose would cause the symptoms; 2) the purpose for using a medicine is to initiate the healing process by stimulating the body's own capacities; and 3) drugs, called remedies, that have undergone a specific pharmaceutical process of many dilutions and vigorous shaking are used.

Although Hahnemann practiced medicine through the 1800s, he had a radical, extraordinary understanding of cancer causation. He recognized a genetic aspect to cancer, the contribution of diet and chronic illnesses to the development of cancer, and the importance of past experiences and mental and emotional states in the initiation of cancer conditions. The concept of individual susceptibility and genetic disposition plays a large role in cancer development, and homeopathy aspires to decrease the individual's susceptibility.

Homeopath practitioners would recommend homeopathy as "an adjunct to conventional treatment for cancer, particularly in cases for which the efficacy of conventional treatment is limited, and as treatment for side effects and peripheral issues that arise during conventional cancer treatment."[3] Homeopathic remedies do not interact adversely with conventional cancer treatment drugs and can be integrated even with the most aggressive cancer protocols.

The evidence is strong for the use of homeopathy in the area of prevention. A practitioner can cull much information about his or her patients during an interview. Who is this patient? What is the nature of his vital force? Does he have an innate susceptibility to diseases such as cancer? How sensitive is he? Will he soak up remedies quickly, and will his body react strongly, or will he be slow in changing? What is his everyday environment like? What is his diet? The answers to these questions will lead to the chosen remedy and correct potency. The chosen remedy will be what homeopaths call "constitutional remedy." It will strengthen the patient's vital force, support him through life challenges, and keep him balanced and the very best he can be.

Pets, like their human guardians, can be stressed. Stress can be physical, or it can be a mental or emotional blow, such as a companion's death. If the stress is too prolonged and severe or the pet is particularly sensitive, the pet may never recover completely, and illness can result. Over time the pet will begin to show symptoms. The reaction to the stress becomes a layer over his innate self, and it is at this level that prescribing begins. In considering any case, the practitioner will weigh any trigger (if there is one), the whole symptom picture (physical, mental, and emotional), and the constitution of the patient.

10

YOUR PET'S DIGESTIVE SYSTEM
AND INTERNAL ORGAN HEALTH

Just as the introduction of antioxidant supplements will change your pet's internal environment for the better, probiotic supplementation will reverse digestion problems and is one of the strongest weapons available in the fight against cancer. Probiotics help the digestive tract in its elimination of toxic substances and waste produced in the body and helps the immune system identify and eliminate viruses and unhealthy bacteria.

Every digestive system needs microflora, the beneficial microorganisms called probiotics. Probiotics are defined as naturally occurring, health-enhancing microorganisms consumed as a food component or as a dietary supplement. The intestinal flora consists of 100 million bacteria from more than 100 species, carrying along with them a variety of enzymes to heal and enhance digestive functions. They do a very important job.

For centuries, people consumed probiotics as part of their food supply in the form of fermented milk; in the same fashion, they probably gave their animals probiotics as well. In 1908, *The Elongation of Life*, by Dr. Elie Metchnikoff, was published; this was the first book to advocate the use of probiotics. It brought the health benefits attributed to the drinking of fermented milk to the world's attention.

Probiotics thrive on lactose and produce lactic acid, which in turn acidifies the colon. These bacteria normalize bowel movements by processing bodily wastes and decreasing the time it takes for waste products to travel through the system. Putrefaction doesn't have the chance to occur, and pathogens can't stick to the walls of the intestines once the intestinal lining is saturated with good bacteria.

That's not all they do. Probiotic replacement is extremely important if there has been damage to the gastrointestinal (GI) tract—damage from stress, surgery, drug therapy, prolonged poor diet, chronic illness, or other factors that can lead to a severe loss of beneficial flora (benign intestinal bacteria). Repair comes from simply replacing the correct flora. A minimum dose of 1 billion bacteria per day is regarded as necessary for a healthy system.

The word "correct" is important. The effectiveness of probiotic supplementation depends on what strains are in the product and the product itself—how it is prepared, processed, and packaged. Some flora strains play a major role in the small intestine, others in the large intestine. Some are found in both areas. A system needs two major strains: the super strains of *Lactobacillus acidophilus* and the various strains of *bifidobacteria.*

Lactobacillus acidophilus colonizes the small intestine and the *bifidobacteria*, the large intestine. They are permanent strains. There are transient strains as well, such as the *bulgaricus* species, one of the world's most powerful beneficial bacteria. Each type works in its own niche. The *acidophilus* strains are grown in milk-based formulas or in dairy-free formulas, such as in a garbanzo bean extract for the lactose-intolerant gut. The others can come in a vegetable oil base. Strains are usually freeze-dried, a process referred to as lyophilizing, a way to preserve their potency and enable them to survive in stomach acid.

Probiotics have been one of the most ignored therapeutic tools of medicine—and, sadly, underutilized. They improve every aspect of digestion and can help heal most problems of the digestive tract. Probiotics play a role in both prevention and treatment of cancer. Chemotherapy agents, radiation, and steroids (the drugs most utilized in conventional pet cancer care) kill the beneficial flora in a pet's digestive tract. Often, the acute result of conventional therapy is diarrhea and loss of appetite, and cachexia results; the long-term result will be poor digestion, malnutrition because of lower metabolism, and absorption of nutrients and eventual nutritional deficiencies.

Without normal microbial populations, the body can't make some of the vitamins it needs. Beneficial flora produces vitamin K, a fat-soluble vitamin manufactured only in the intestinal tract in the presence of intestinal flora.

No flora, no vitamin K. Vitamin K helps to prevent internal bleeding and hemorrhaging and contributes to the formation of the blood-clotting factor prothrombin. Probiotics also help to produce the B family. Every B vitamin is a part of an important team, part of whose work is to prevent cancer by disintegrating tumor cells, altering their membrane, and preventing chromosome damage.

Beneficial flora slows down the body's natural aging process, supports the host's immune system responses, and plays a big part in the body's ability to resist infection. Japanese researchers working with the elderly found that daily dietary supplementation of probiotics, as in cultured milk products, prevented constipation and a host of geriatric diseases. Impressively, *acidophilus* supplementation in patients suppressed liver tumors by 65 percent, particularly those caused by *E. coli*, *S. faecalis*, and *C. paraputrificum*, which reside in the intestines.

Lactobacillus bulgaricus, the flora that resides in both the small and the large intestine, is the most potent producer of much-needed lactic acid, which lowers the pH in the colon and forms a hostile environment for disease-causing bacteria. By establishing a pH of 5.0, it creates a desirable environment for all the other *bifidobacteria* to thrive in. *Bulgaricus* produces anticarcinogenic compounds; it helps increase the number of leukocytes, particularly the desirable T-lymphocytes; it stimulates antitumor activity through macrophage production (cells in the first line of defense against foreign particles entering the body); it enhances the production of immunoglobulin A, an antibody always on the lookout for invading microorganisms; and it regulates peristaltic action in the intestinal tract, and, as the *bulgaricus* cells die, the resident strains feed on their remains, ensuring their own survival and growth.

Probiotics help to destroy a huge spectrum of disease-causing pathogens just by being present in sufficient numbers to crowd them out. They inhibit the growth of *Salmonella*, *E. coli*, and *Shigella*, all of which cause gastroenteritis or virulent diarrhea. They produce a fatty acid that helps ward off fungi and yeast overloads, such as *Candida*, in the intestines. Chemotherapy agents and steroids that are often given in tandem with anticancer agents often cause a yeast overload.

The loss of good flora and the development of intestinal inflammation can lead to cancer. The intestinal tract is the source of all nutrient access, and if not working properly, the intestinal wall is covered with hardened waste and colonies of harmful pathogens. The average human stores many pounds of old fecal matter (as can cats and dogs), and this old fecal matter is an ideal breeding ground for problems such as inflammation and the situation known as "leaky gut syndrome"—the dumping of foreign particles from the intestines into the body. The liver filters out through the colon, but a plugged gut can't handle the toxins. An added burden is put on the liver. The lymphatic system is also compromised; lymph fluid, which collects the heavy metals and pesticides and drug residues stored in the body's tissues, can't eliminate them if the gut is plugged or sluggish.

Lack of beneficial flora can alter cellular RNA and DNA blueprints. In the least-worst case, the abnormal growth of bacterial and viral infections creates a parasitic overload, which is called dysbiosis. In either case, the mucosal walls must be repaired. That can be accomplished by replacing the missing flora with more of the best intestinal flora, along with essential fatty acids, the amino acid glutamine, the antioxidant enzymes superoxide dismutase and catalase, and glutathione.

THE TROUBLE WITH YEAST

The most common form of bacterial and fungal overgrowth is yeast, or *Candida*. Candidiasis affects almost every part of the body, showing up in a wide range of symptoms. It can cause abdominal pain, noise, gas, and bloating. In the mouth, it can cause burning, spotted tongue, soreness in the corners, canker sores, bad breath, and gum problems. On the skin, it causes hives, itchy fungal infections, acne, and chronic rashes. In the respiratory system, it has been known to swell membranes, producing a nagging cough, congestion, and allergic reactions. In the nose, it clogs sinuses. In the urinary tract, it causes kidney and bladder infections. In females, it can cause hormonal imbalances, vaginitis, and infertility. *Candida* toxins also integrate with hormones to alter brain and nervous system functions and can be the underlying cause of systemic problems of low energy, irritability, aching joints, anxiety, and headaches—in other words, a litany of ill-defined problems.

If your pet—especially your dog—has been on steroids, hormone replacement drugs, immunosuppressive drugs, or chemotherapy agents; has had a chronic viral, bacterial, or parasitic infestation; or has been on poor-quality food (especially food loaded with additives) for most of his life, he is likely to suffer from candidiasis and is a good candidate for probiotic supplementation. Moreover, any animal that has been put on one or more courses of a broad-spectrum antibiotic probably has little good flora left in his GI system. Antibiotics are often recommended after surgery and if the pet has developed an infection from his stay in the hospital. The GI system is consequently unprotected, its doors open to malabsorption, dysbiosis, leaky gut syndrome, irritable bowel syndrome, and more. At a minimum, the imbalance between the good and bad intestinal bacteria leaves the animal vulnerable to additional infections and *Candida*.

My program to eliminate *Candida* is an aggressive one. You start with what I call the avoidance part. For one month, avoid giving the dog the following:

- Any product with refined white flour, including biscuit treats
- Any multivitamin except one that is guaranteed to be yeast free
- Foods such as cheese
- Fruit because of its natural sugars
- Meats that have been cured, smoked, preserved, pickled, or otherwise processed
- The drug Myostatin, which is often prescribed as an antifungal but which causes a resurgence of yeast within four weeks after treatment with it ends
- Dried legumes (these may contain hidden mold)

While avoiding the above, begin feeding the dog the following on a daily basis:

- Biscuits or treats made from whole grains
- Small amounts (one or two teaspoons) of goat cheese a few times a week
- 100 milligrams of vitamin B complex
- Grape seed extract (either one-quarter teaspoon or a capsule a day, usually about 60 milligrams)
- A small amount (one-quarter teaspoon) of cold-pressed, virgin olive oil drizzled on his food
- *L. bulgaricus* powder (one-eighth teaspoon) every day about 10 minutes before food (gradually increase the dose to one teaspoon a day; this can be mixed into a small amount of good, unflavored, live-cultured yogurt)

- *L. acidophilus* powder (two and a half teaspoons) before meals and in yogurt
- *E. faecium* powder (two teaspoons) before food (each of these flora addresses a specific part of the GI system; they are the proper ones for dogs and cats)
- Good, unflavored, live-cultured yogurt (one or two tablespoons), which can be mixed into food
- Organically grown meat or poultry, cooked at home and making up about 60 percent of the meal
- Easily digestible vegetables, such as sweet potato, squashes, and carrots, cooked
- Grains, such as those that are soy or rice based

You now have a good plan to begin with; when combined with probiotics, it will work wonders for the pet that is suffering GI problems after months on chemotherapy and may develop a problem in tolerating various foods. With probiotics, bowels will be normalized. Moreover, the probiotics will also stop any diarrhea-causing bacteria from proliferating and robbing the body of nutrients. Probiotics also increase the bioavailability of calcium, helping to prevent bone loss and the consequent degeneration in the density and strength of the bone matrix.

Probiotics are present in live-cultured, unflavored yogurt; this food is a good adjunct to a diet. But it is not necessarily the solution to a probiotic deficiency. First, there are many brands of yogurt on the market; however, many popular products incorporate inexpensive, poor-quality, or dead flora, which are useless, and the flavored varieties often contain sugars, which can actually feed a yeast problem. Probiotics should be sold by themselves and should state on the label the "viable cell count," along with the identity of the living bacterial strains. Look for the most powerful strains of each species. Products should list a genus or species such as *L. acidophilus*, *L. bulgaricus*, or *L. casei*. In the case of *bifidobacteria*, the label should read *bifidus*, *longum*, *infantis*, and so on. Does the product contain a minimum total of 2 billion to 3 billion microorganisms per dose? Is the expiration date far enough in the future to be practical? And has the product been refrigerated to keep it from losing its usefulness? These are vital considerations.

The liquid culturing medium called the supernatant is an essential part of the product and is as important as the live bacteria itself. Many probiotic manufacturers avoid the supernatant when they freeze-dry their product, as it can add substantially to the production cost. The supernatant contains by-products produced by the microorganisms and bacteria, which make the product more effective by up to 50 percent and guarantee a longer shelf life.

Some products have additional ingredients, such as vitamins and minerals, as an extended benefit. But a minimum of bacteria added to a multi-vitamin or mineral supplement will probably not have enough viable cells to achieve flora replacement. Digestive tracts need multiple strains and plenty of them.

Probiotics are sold in capsule, powder, and gel forms. When you decide to put your pet on a program, you can start off with one dose a day, 10 to 15 minutes before food, for a week. If needed, you can dose him twice a day. Starting with more frequent doses restores colonies faster. Once the replacement flora are established, the dosage can be dropped down to two or three times a week. You can mix the powders into unflavored, live-cultured yogurt and mix in a small amount of food for a between-meals snack. Always store probiotics in the refrigerator.

CLEANING THE BODY INTERNALLY

When you or your pet's groomer scrubs him up, he not only looks great but feels great, too. If he had an internal bath periodically, he would have a very healthy inside as well. Health is impossible without clean organs, such as the liver and kidneys, and clean systems, such as the blood and lymph systems. Periodically, all these parts should be cleansed, detoxed, and repaired.

Let's take the liver first. It's impossible for a pet to go through months of ingesting highly toxic drugs such as anticancer agents and have a healthy liver. To repair and rebuild the liver, we must remove the toxic waste accumulated over months and get bile flowing freely again. We need to reduce any inflammation and regenerate damaged cells. This is a really big cleaning.

Next to the skin, the liver is the largest organ in the body. In some ways, it is the most important organ and often the last to be considered when it comes to cleaning. The liver is involved in over 200 separate functions: it regulates fat stores; cleans the blood; neutralizes poisons;

helps in using and recycling proteins; manages blood chemistry; aids digestion by producing bile and enzymes; helps resist infections by producing immune factors; stores vitamins, minerals, and sugars; controls cholesterol; maintains hormone balances; and, through all this, is able to heal its own damaged tissue.

How does the liver become toxic? Diet is one factor: eating too much protein overstresses the liver. Metabolizing protein takes a lot of work; the greater the consumption, the more work the liver has to do. Too much carbohydrate and fat in the diet is also difficult on the liver. The body converts excess simple carbohydrates into triglycerides, which, in turn, are stored in the liver as fat. A fatty liver can't perform its duties.

All the medicinal drugs your pet has been given in his lifetime have to be processed and eliminated through the liver. Some of these drugs cause inflammation of liver tissue. Once inflamed, the liver can't filter; the organ plugs up, becomes more inflamed, and eventually hardens. This is called cirrhosis.

Everything your pet eats and breathes in is purified by the liver. That means that all the toxins, heavy metals, and environmental pollutants will pass through the liver. The liver does indeed carry a heavy burden and usually receives little or no reward for all its work. Perhaps the time has come to do something for it.

If you help your pet's liver, it will astound you in its thanks. The liver has a great ability to regenerate itself, but it needs your help to do so. A detox diet is an excellent starting place. During a detox, the liver is purging all the fats, cholesterol deposits, gallstones, poisons, drug residues, and just about every toxic waste it has been holding on to for years. The diet goes like this: for five days, your dog or cat eats only a raw vegetable and sprout salad topped with a dressing of fresh, cold-pressed olive oil and lemon, two or more times a day. He must abstain from all other solid food. Make a drink for him of fresh fruit and fresh vegetables and include cooked beets in the vegetable version. Snacks of fresh vegetables or a fruit smoothie can be included.

Cups of potassium broth should be offered every day in lieu of water. Take the peelings from several potatoes—up to one-quarter cup for most dogs to one-half cup if the dog is a giant breed. The outside of the potato is one of the highest plant sources of potassium. Don't use the inside of the potato. Add other well-chopped vegetables, such as carrots, celery, whole beets, and fresh greens, to four cups of clean, filtered water and simmer for

40 to 60 minutes in a covered pan over low heat. Strain out the vegetables, cool, and leave it for the dog or cat to drink throughout the day. Keep any remainder in a glass container in the refrigerator.

Treating the liver to a good flush begins the detox part. The use of herbal mixes is essential. You can mix your own blend of herbs if bought as tinctures or buy a liver flush detox mix. Key herbs for a mix are dandelion, parsley root, and thistles. Dandelion is one of the strongest tonics for the liver; adding equal parts of three or four other herbs, such as milk thistle, artichoke, burdock root, horsetail herb, and parsley root, enhances the effect. This liver detox tincture is a good place to include an antiparasitic herb, like wormwood or black walnut. The dose is two droppers full, three times a day for an adult, large-size dog; half the dose for a medium-size dog; and one-third the dose for a small dog or cat. During the first five days, you may see what looks like small green or black stones (bile) or tiny white crystals (cholesterol) pass in the stool. Since the detox has to pass through the intestines, you need to add glutathione once a day to aid the elimination process through the intestines.

The body's blood supply is filled with just as many impurities as the liver, including too many fats and toxic heavy metals. The blood of cancer patients is often characterized by hyperviscosity and hypercoagulability, conditions that help cancer cells adhere to the microcapillaries and decrease permeability and the penetration of medications. This change in the blood causes sludge buildup in the arteries. Since the blood replaces itself every 120 days, it makes sense to freshen it up.

Cleaning the blood begins with herbs. A good herbal mix contains some or all of the following: red clover blossoms, burdock root, chaparral, periwinkle, and goldenseal. These are blended together; a dose of one dropper full, twice a day, will do the job. (A large animal can take one and a half droppers full, a small animal one-half a dropper.) You can purchase a dropper in any pharmacy.

Another important addition is oral chelation, which is based on the amino acid cysteine, malic acid, or cilantro herb. All of these chelators will grab on to heavy metals, such as aluminum, lead, and mercury, in the cardiovascular system and pull them out of the body. By removing heavy metals, chelation therapy reduces the production of free radicals in the bloodstream and their consequent scarring of the arterial walls.

If you decide to make a cilantro chelator, process one cup of packed-fresh cilantro and six tablespoons of olive oil in a blender until the cilantro is chopped. Add one clove of garlic, one-half cup of almonds, and two tablespoons of lemon juice. Blend together. Your pet can be given a teaspoon of this mix every day for three weeks.

The pH of the blood is very important. The body has a whole range of pH levels: blood pH is slightly alkaline, saliva is slightly alkaline, the stomach is strongly acidic, the intestines are strongly alkaline, and urine is acidic. But of all the pH levels in the body, the most crucial is that of the blood. Since every cell requires oxygen, a slightly alkaline blood supply maintains optimum oxygen availability. An acidic blood supply binds up the available oxygen, and cells suffocate. The pH balance comes primarily from food. All meats, fish, poultry, eggs, dairy, cooked grains, and refined sugars are acid-forming foods. Fresh fruit and vegetables are alkaline forming and help the body keep its proper overall pH.

Changing the pH depends in large part on changing the diet. Eliminating acids is handled through neutralizing them with minerals such as calcium, magnesium, and potassium. If there are not enough minerals to do the work, the body will steal them from anywhere it can. Blood must not become too acidic; if it does, the body will begin leaching calcium from the bones as one solution. Osteoporosis is preferable to death.

It's a good idea to test your pet's pH levels on a regular basis. You can buy pH paper that is specifically designed to test saliva at most health food stores. Make sure to test before brushing your pet's teeth or before he eats. If the pH tests below 7.0, you should get aggressive in terms of alkalizing.

Next on the list is the intestinal tract. Your pet's "internal bath" is incomplete without an intestinal cleaning out. A cleaning will remove old fecal matter and water from the colon, and it will get rid of all heavy metals and drug residues that have accumulated in the waste. The colon musculature will strengthen as a result of cleaning, and damage from inflammation in either intestine can be repaired as well. A cleaning will help eliminate the presence of polyps and other abnormal growths that have been allowed to flourish because of an unhealthy intestinal environment. In addition, a cleaning will allow you to replenish and rebuild the various friendly bacterial cultures that belong there.

A good cleaning is a two-step process: use herbs to pull out old fecal matter and scrape off impacted sludge and then add probiotics at an aggressive level of two or three times a day. The friendly bacteria will colonize every space on the walls, leaving no area open to pathogen recolonization. The herbs will stimulate the muscular movement of the colon and disinfect, soothe, and heal mucous membrane linings. Look for a formula that contains organic herbs such as aloe, senna, cascara sagrada, barberry root, ginger root, and fennel. Or make your own formula, choosing two or three, depending on the issues you want to address. For example, constipation can be treated with cascara sagrada coupled with aloe.

You may need a stronger purifier and cleanser if your pet's intestines have never been detoxed. A purifier should include marshmallow root and psyllium seeds and/or husks. Fiber in the diet is an absolute necessity. A good source is ground, organic, flaxseed meal: one and a half tablespoons for a big dog, one teaspoon for a medium-size dog, one-half teaspoon for a small dog, and one-quarter teaspoon for the average-size cat. Include foods such as squash or pumpkin and apple slices with the peel.

Your pet's life span is directly related to how well his own detoxification organs are working. A healthy colon is one of his body's first lines of defense. A clean, peak-performing liver; purified blood; and a slightly alkaline pH are other baselines for health.

The last recommendation is a fast. Your dog or cat can easily fast one or two days a month or a few times a year. When you deprive his body of food, it begins to consume itself to survive. Being geared to survive, the body chooses to consume damaged cells and toxic cells first, saving the healthiest for later. The body is actually healing itself. You have diverted the energy used to process food into an energy that repairs and rebuilds. Provide plenty of filtered water, and, if you wish, you can allow fruit juices or vegetable broth as well. You can also provide for his basic nutrient needs by adding spirulina and chlorella to the program.

THE ROLE OF FIBER

Changing the internal environment has to include fiber. A very important part of what is missing from human diets is fiber. Records from 1909 through 1979 show a 28 percent decrease in our consumption of fiber. This decrease in crude fiber consumption supports the hypothesis that decreases in fiber intake are linked to increases in colon cancer (along with colitis, hemorrhoids, diverticulosis, and chronic constipation). By avoiding fiber, we are giving our bodies permission to develop serious problems—and we are doing the same thing to our pets.

There are several basic classifications of fiber; most of these are found in food. Everyone has heard of bran—oat bran and rice bran being the most popular—which is the broken coat of the seed of cereal grain. It is often sifted out in processing. Pectin, another common form of fiber, is found in apples, bananas, beets, cabbage, citrus fruits, and some dried legumes. Pectin slows the absorption of food through the system; it also helps lower cholesterol, reduces the risk of gallstones, and removes unwanted metals and toxins. Cellulose is a fiber found in the outer layer of vegetables and fruits. It helps to remove cancer-causing substances from the colon walls. Giving some apple slices, part of a pear, some broccoli or green beans with a meal, and carrots for a snack will provide an animal's daily cellulose. Cellulose's relative, hemicellulose fiber, is another complex carbohydrate that absorbs water, relieves constipation, and prevents colon cancer. Leafy green vegetables, beans, cabbage, and peppers are the chief vegetable providers of this fiber; apples and bananas are the main fruit sources. Lignins are good for lowering cholesterol levels and helping to prevent gallstones. Good vegetable sources include green beans, carrots, peas, and tomatoes; good fruit sources are peaches and strawberries.

Fiber has little or no food value; it isn't digested or absorbed. It passes through the digestive tract, accumulating liquid, and swells up to provide a good amount of soft bulk to stools, helping to stimulate bowel contractions. Regular bowel movements are an important mechanism for removing toxins. Fiber also dilutes levels of fat metabolites associated with the action of carcinogens.

The apparent protective effect of dietary fiber against colon cancer comes partly from the action of intestinal bacteria on the fiber, producing a by-product called butyric acid. Butyric acid induces cell differentiation: the ability to acquire the functions of mature, normal cells. When abnormal cells are exposed to differentiating agents, such as butyric acid, they lose their ability to proliferate madly; butyric acid is also known to induce cancer cell death (apoptosis). All cells are programmed to die either at old age or under circumstances where cell death benefits the host. Apoptosis is an orderly method of removing old, damaged, or otherwise unwanted cells and plays a big role in limiting tumor growth.

Fiber reduces the concentrations of carcinogens in the stool. Some chemicals, while not directly causing cancer, are categorized as cancer causing because they break down into carcinogenic metabolites. Fiber plus beneficial flora destroy carcinogenic metabolites.

Fiber-rich diets may reduce the incidence of breast cancer by reducing estrogen levels. Estrogen compounds are made in the liver and empty into the intestines through the bile. Fiber suppresses the ability of fecal bacteria to recycle estrogen, binds it to the stool, and facilitates the elimination of estrogen. In one large Canadian study of 56,837 women, those who consumed high amounts of fiber had a 30 percent reduction in the risk of breast cancer compared to those who consumed low amounts of fiber.[1]

Fiber reduces serum cholesterol and pulls fats from the body. Dogs can develop high cholesterol levels; if obese, the animal's body will store the fats as toxins in fatty tissue. When a dog is put on a diet and starts to lose weight, the body releases some of these toxins; he now needs the protective help of a greater intake of fiber, water, and antioxidants.

Fiber comes in a great diversity of appearances, textures, colors, and flavors. You don't need to use chemical fiber additions or harsh purgatives to get the same results you would from natural fiber sources.

THE SURGICAL SUPPORT PROGRAM

The following information focuses on how to help the pet who has already been diagnosed with cancer. The most-well-defined and straightforward-to-treat cases are those where surgery is indicated and the tumor can be completely removed. Nothing more needs to be done on that level. But you can ensure better results by taking some additional steps before the procedure.

If the surgery can be put off for two or three weeks, you can initiate a preparedness program that will build up your pet's strength before the operation. This strategy can also aid in making his biochemistry as hostile as possible to the spread of cancer cells from the original tumor. In addition, the plan will strengthen his natural defenses against infection and reduce postoperative pain and swelling.

Let's begin with preparing the patient for the ordeal. You have a choice among several traditional Chinese medicine herbal formulas. One such formula, called All-Inclusive Great Tonifying Herbal Formula, contains several of the most effective herbs in the herbal pharmacopeia, and its aim is to build up the body's resistance to any unforeseen problems. This formula has traditionally been administered to patients in weakened conditions, including those going into surgery with chronic illnesses—which is what cancer is. It alleviates fatigue, loss of appetite, pale mucosa, and dry skin and, in general, will nourish the energy and blood of the animal. This formula's biological impact includes enhancing certain white blood cells, among them phagocytes, T-cells, and natural killer cells, and has general antitumor effects when combined with surgery. In the case of leukemia, it protects against the ill effects of anticancer drugs, radiation-induced immunosuppression, and bone marrow toxicity. The formula is especially beneficial to elderly animals. It can be given on a daily basis for two to three weeks before scheduled surgery. It comes in capsule and granule form.

I would also recommend a Chinese herbal formula called *Yunnan Baiyao*. This herbal treatment is a must just before surgery, as it is the best all-around formula to stop traumatic bleeding. It halts hemorrhaging almost immediately and prevents infection. Interestingly, this formula both stops bleeding and removes blood clots, a seeming contradiction. As the bleeding stops, blood tends to congeal in the wound, blocking normal circulation and preventing the wound from healing properly. *Yunnan Baiyao* maintains normal circulation, flushing out pus and congealed blood. Flesh regenerates with minimal scarring. The formula can be taken internally if there is suspicion of internal hemorrhage or to prevent or stop infection. This can be helpful for head injuries where there may be bruising or bleeding of the brain. In these cases, it is vital that any bleeding or excessive clotting be stopped.

The formula is effective when applied directly to open and infected wounds. If the wound is bleeding, sprinkle the powder form into the wound and apply pressure. Once the bleeding has stopped, clean or irrigate the wound, then cover it with a paste of water and herbs and bandage it. In the case of suppurating wounds, it's better to just sprinkle the powder around the area and cover it. Simultaneous internal and external use of the formula helps the flesh to regenerate.

Yunnan Baiyao is helpful in postsurgical healing even when it comes to less invasive surgery. In this case, wait two or three days after the procedure before giving your pet the capsule form twice a day. Open wounds need to be treated correctly to prevent scarring. Once the scar is closed but still red and tender, apply pearl powder (made from real pearls) by making it into a paste with water. Then cover the area. This should be repeated several times a day while the scar is healing.

Yunnan Baiyao falls under the category of first aid. Americans discovered it in Vietnam during the war there; they found capsules or vials of this white powder on wounded and dead Vietcong and North Vietnamese soldiers. These men had been supplied with the medicine and instructed to use it in cases of gunshot wounds, knife wounds, and so on. Each blister pack of capsules and each vial of powder came with a red pill; the pill was to be taken only in case of serious injuries, such as stab or gunshot wounds. For our purposes, the powder form of the formula is easier to use externally and the capsule form easier to give internally. Give your pet a capsule or one-quarter teaspoon of powder the night before and on the morning of surgery.

Preparedness also involves careful scrutiny of any tests or blood work done on the pet. The results will tell us if the cat or dog is able to go forward with the desired plan. Three years ago, I saw a beautiful Malamute named Bertha that, despite several attempts at insemination, remained infertile. Although this case has no bearing on cancer, it does illustrate the point I want to make. When I looked over her blood tests, I noted that Bertha had a suppressed immune system. Her white blood cell activity was almost nonexistent. Bertha had previously been taken to a well-known holistic veterinarian who had put the dog on several herbal formulas for infertility. I pointed out that with almost no immunity, a pregnancy was next to impossible. Even if Bertha did somehow conceive, one would have to ask if the pregnancy would be viable, could she carry to term, and what the health of the offspring would be. My advice was to get her blood count back to normal and then move forward. After herbal and supplemental treatment aimed at immune system enhancement, Bertha had three beautiful puppies.

Some animals do not react well to the drugs used for anesthesia. For these cases, there are homeopathic remedies. Phosphorus is the first one to try. I was called about a dog in Vermont that could not come out of anesthesia without having a seizure. Phosphorus is what I recommended to treat any such sequela. Phosphorus can be rubbed on the gums, on the foot pads, and inside the ear flaps if the animal is unconscious. This should be repeated several times until the animal awakens peacefully. This remedy should also be used if your pet appears listless or disoriented, is nauseous or vomits, or shows any signs of ill effects of drugs, especially an anesthetic.

Arnica in homeopathic form is the remedy of choice for soft-tissue injury. Arnica is indicated when the patient's condition worsens as a result of moving, jarring, or even touching the injured part. It promotes healing, helps control bleeding and swelling, and prevents infections at the wound site. Any bruise or injury to the body, with or without discoloration, heals faster with this remedy. If there is severe bruising and discoloration, Arnica given internally and Arnica gel or ointment used externally works wonders.

Any stressful incident, such as an accident, surgery, dental work, or birthing, should be treated with Arnica for fast, complete healing. Give three pellets of Arnica 200c right before surgery, three pellets after surgery is finished, and three pellets later in the day or before sleep.

Another great remedy for postsurgical problems is Ledum. Ledum is a big help in the case of persistent pain, swelling, severe bruising, or trauma at the sight of an injection. Ledum is a combination of Arnica and Hypericum and works on wounds caused by sharp objects such as needles. It is a superb follow-on treatment to Arnica.

If the animal goes into shock, is morbidly afraid, or shakes uncontrollably, homeopathic Aconitum is the answer. A dose of three or four pellets of 30c or 200c every 15 minutes for a total of four doses will make a big difference. An animal that is in shock or unconscious can be administered any homeopathic remedy by crushing or melting the substance in a very small amount of water and applying this to the gums, ear flaps, or foot pads several times at 15-minute intervals.

Calendula ointment helps speed up the healing of surgical wounds without complications. The ointment should be applied to the wound twice a day after the dressing has been removed; then the wound is re-covered. Calendula in pellet form is also advised for internal healing; the dose is five pellets of 6c or 200c, two to three times a day for three weeks.

If there has been trauma to internal organs, such as the stomach, liver, or spleen; if the pain is quite deep; or as a later follow-up to Arnica, particularly if there are lumps in the area of the trauma, the homeopathic remedy Bellis is the answer. Bellis should follow the use of Arnica when symptoms clearly indicate intense soreness or if Arnica has failed. The remedy Hypericum is indicated when there has been injury to the nerves; this could be trauma to the peripheral or spinal nerves. Both remedies should be used at 200c potency, if possible, otherwise 30c. The dose is usually three or four pellets, dry, two times a day.

If your pet has been given antibiotics before or after surgery or has been on steroids for his cancer, it will be necessary to undo the negative effects of these drugs, particularly their impact on the gastrointestinal system. Adding probiotics (good bacteria) to the plan will undo the loss of beneficial intestinal bacteria and prevent diarrhea, loss of appetite, or the growth of *Candida* or a yeast overload. Probiotics for animals are completely different strains from those for humans, although there are a few human forms that can be very good in some cases.

You can buy a number of these herbal and homeopathic remedies on your own. Just be sure that they are of the best quality. Buy from companies with good reputations and consistent quality control. Many of these remedies, of course, can be obtained from a practitioner. Together, you can set up a program tailored to your pet's particular set of problems and needs.

You can begin to implement the next steps as soon as your pet has clearly recovered:

- Honsho #48 All-Inclusive Great Tonifying Herbal Formula comes in capsule and granule forms. If you can pill your pet, use the capsule; if not, you can put granules in the food or in a chicken broth solution or in baby food. Dosage is as follows: one packet twice a day or two capsules twice a day for a medium-size dog; one packet a day divided into one-half doses or one capsule twice a day for a small dog or cat. Birds can be given a capsule a day or half a packet: sprinkle over foods such as vegetables and add a tiny amount to the drinking water. Large animals need three to five packets, or six capsules, a day. Herbs can be given with or without food.
- *Yunnan Baiyao* comes in capsule and powder forms. The powder is used primarily externally, covering the lesion, wound, or incision. As a preventive measure, one capsule can be given the night before and on the morning of the surgery. Additional doses can be given, if needed, after surgery.
- Probiotics for pets come in either powder, capsule, or gel forms and are given on an empty stomach once or twice a day. Buy only if the product has been refrigerated and keep it in the refrigerator at home.
- Homeopathic remedies come in varying potencies; the most common one sold in stores is the 30c. These pellets should be given dry on an empty stomach, or, if necessary, they can be crushed and added to a very small amount of water before administering. A dose of three or four pellets, given or applied every 15 minutes in acute cases for a total of four doses, is the usual strategy; in chronic cases, three pellets, dry, once a day, is the norm. The ointment form is applied two to three times a day and, even if licked off, is not harmful. Higher doses need to be supplied by a professional.

For sequella to surgery, see Appendix C.

12

THE CHEMOTHERAPY
SUPPORT PROGRAM: PAIRINGS

The goal of cancer treatment is to eliminate the cancer. Surgery may remove all visible cancer, but some microscopic cancer cells may remain in the body. This is why oncologists frequently recommend further treatment—chemotherapy and/or radiation therapy. The purpose of these therapies is to keep the disease from returning. Despite their ability to be effective in many ways, both therapies are harsh and toxic; however, natural compounds paired with these conventional therapies make them more tolerable and less risky and promote faster recovery, and, importantly, a support program of alternative medicine exceeds expectations by years. While you are unlikely to have heard of them previously, the constituents of these pairings—called cytoprotectants—are chosen based on research and clinical experience. You need not fear that they represent a "throw-anything-at-the-problem" approach.

Cancer cells, by their nature, resist being killed. Solid tumors, especially, can acquire this resistance, responding to treatment initially but then recurring later, sometimes more strongly than ever. In such instances, tumor cells that were vulnerable to the chemotherapy or radiation were killed, but a critical mass of resistant cells may have survived. These now have a clear field to multiply and make further treatment more difficult. Acquired drug resistance remains one of the biggest barriers to true remission. If your pet is about to undergo chemotherapy or radiation, consider working with a holistic or complementary and alternative practitioner to help make those therapies more effective:

- *Reduced L-glutathione:* This amino acid enhances chemotherapy drug sensitivity, particularly on glioblastoma and glioma cell lines. It prevents bladder damage and hematuria (blood in the urine) when coupled with the chemotherapy agent cyclophosphamide. Glutathione reduces the toxicity of the drug cisplatin and protects the nervous system through the course of the therapy. The amino acid is often used to prevent peripheral neurotoxicity and has demonstrated a positive outcome in 73 percent of cases versus 63 percent with conventional treatment alone. Evidence indicates that glutathione supplementation is capable of switching cell death from necrosis to apoptosis. (Necrotic death leaves all its "garbage" behind, but apoptosis is a real reversion from abnormal to normal differentiation within the cell.[1])
- *N-acetylcysteine:* This amino acid enhances interleukin-2's cancer-killing effect. It assists in various detoxification processes and reduces the toxic side effects of conventional treatments. It is a precursor for the production of glutathione.
- *Astragalus:* This is a major herb of the traditional Chinese medicine pharmacopeia. In 34 clinical trials, this herb in formula combinations resulted in a 34 percent improvement in the response to chemotherapy and a 33 percent reduction in the risk of death from the therapy. Research has shown it to be a potent immune system stimulant. I often recommend it, formulated with other immune system enhancers, after conventional treatment, for long-term protection.[2]
- *Quercetin:* This bioflavonoid reduces cisplatin toxicity in renal (kidney) cells and potentiates the effects of Adriamycin and tamoxifen drugs. It lowers the pH inside the cancer cell and decreases the likelihood that tumor cells will proliferate or metastasize.[3]
- *Gingko biloba:* This phytonutrient, coupled with 5-FU (fluorouracil), enhances the chemotherapy effect. Some practitioners use this herb as a blood cleanser and to improve circulation. A study at Loma Linda University found that an extract of the herb is highly effective in curtailing the free radical damage that naturally accompanies anticancer activity. (More on free radicals coming up soon.) Gingko can dramatically lessen the damage to normal cells that is typically associated with the chemotherapy agent Adriamycin.[4] If your pet has had radiation treat-

ments, consider gingko supplementation, a 40-milligram tablet once a day after radiation has ended. Radiation makes the body form oxidizing compounds that circulate in the body and cause chromosome damage.

- *Ginseng:* Studies on toxin-induced cancers show that animals receiving ginseng have a 75 percent lower rate of liver cancer and a 29 percent lower rate of lung cancer than animals that did not receive this herb.[5]

- *Ganoderma:* Ganoderma mushroom is one of a handful of medicinal mushrooms that have potent powers for both treatment and prevention. It has been seen in research and clinical trials to regress the size of tumors by as much as 89 percent. One study found that after 28 days of daily dosing with ganoderma, average tumor weight was down to 0.6 grams; the average weight of untreated tumors after the same period of time was 4.5 grams. In other words, tumors of the same or close to the same weight, within a designated time period, that were treated with ganoderma shrank significantly, while tumors not treated with ganoderma grew significantly. Laboratory tests show that combinations of this mushroom with related medicinal mushrooms activate the entire spectrum of the immune system. If omega-3 (an essential fatty acid) is added to the treatment plan, the mixture produces a particularly strong antitumor effect.[6]

- *Curcumin, or turmeric:* This herb works on squamous cell skin cancers, ulcerating oral cancers, and colon cancer. One study focusing on patients with skin cancer or ulcerating oral cancer who had not responded to conventional therapies showed a significant reduction in the size of their cancerous lesions after treatment with curcumin as well as decreased itching, pain, odor, and drainage. Turmeric hits at least 45 molecules that allow malignant cells to proliferate.

- *Silymarin:* As one main ingredient of the herb milk thistle, silymarin helps protect the liver and gallbladder by detoxifying these organs from the free radicals produced by chemotherapy. It enhances the chemotherapy effect of doxorubicin, cisplatin, and Taxol.[7]

- *Coenzyme Q10:* Some research has shown that using coenzyme Q10 can cause regression of tumors in advanced breast cancer. Usually, this nutrient is added to prevent cardiotoxicity and subsequent damage to heart tissue from chemotherapy agents.[8]

- *Medicinal mushrooms:* Medicinal mushrooms are classified as "host defense potentiators." Used in conjunction with chemotherapy agents, these mushrooms decrease common side effects, such as pain, nausea, and fatigue, by up to 90 percent. The group includes reishi, maitake, ganoderma, cordyceps, and shiitake. They can provide protection to healthy cells from invasion by nearby cancerous ones. They can also increase the production of interleukin-1 and -2.[9]

- *Resveratrol:* This extract of red wine hits 34 molecules that allow malignant cells to metastasize.
- *Vitamin E:* This vitamin protects the nerves and kidneys and reduces the risk of inner-ear damage that may result from chemotherapy. Vitamin E is helpful in protecting against the toxic effects of the therapy.
- *Alpha lipoic acid, glutamine, acetyl-L-carnitine, and vitamin B6:* This combination reduces weakness and numbness due to peripheral neuropathy.

Clinically, patients treated with phytonutrients have twice the survival advantage of those who aren't. In one study of liver cirrhosis, a risk factor for liver cancer, the half of the study population of 260 patients who were treated with phytonutrients along with conventional drugs had a higher survival rate than the patients taking conventional drugs alone. After a five-year follow-up, 78 percent of the patients in the combined phytonutrient program were still alive, compared to 68 percent in the pharmaceutical-only group.[10]

Choose your supplements to meet your particular goals. If your pet is crashing after chemotherapy, your goal has to be free radical mop-up; utilize a rich, herbal formula to build up blood and energy. If your pet develops burns or lesions from radiation therapy, your goal will be met by employing herbal treatment, such as homeopathic calendula ointment or DMSO externally, to heal the wounds as well as deal with the accompanying free radical damage.

The idea of a support program via alternative therapies can't be overemphasized. Of course, the varied approaches to helping our pets have to be weighed against the costs and expectations involved. Costs include your outlay of time and energy as well as the financial investment involved in adopting and maintaining such a program. There are many possibilities. Will this type of a program meet your expectations? Does the chosen program take into consideration a comprehensive view of the entire body as opposed to focusing on just one narrow part? Will the program lead to any negative problems in the future? And, as time goes by, does the original plan continue to be appropriate? The information that follows will help you make the right choice for you and your pet.

13

THE PATIENT SUPPORT PROGRAM: CHINESE HERBAL MEDICINE

Conventional veterinary care for cancer left Ebenezer, a cocker spaniel, with multiple issues. The dog had been diagnosed with melanoma and subsequently was treated with surgery, chemotherapy, and adjunctive drugs—steroids and antibiotics. He was given a survival time of possibly two months regardless of therapy. When I met Ebenezer, he had bloody, itchy, smelly oozing lesions over his body and his ears and one large lesion that covered much of a front paw, causing him a great deal of distress. His owner, Michelle, and I discussed options and developed a multifaceted treatment plan. We started with soaks for his ears and paw. These soaks were herb based; the major ingredient was the herb Astragalus. We made a program of herbs aimed at helping to shrink the tumor and to clear up the smelly discharge and the yeast buildup created by the antibiotics, steroids, and chemotherapy agents. His owner upgraded his diet to a mix of chicken and vegetables and had him take daily doses of probiotics. Ebenezer also had acupuncture treatments once a week for a month.

The dog's skin improved remarkably, and the unpleasant odor disappeared. He enjoyed his food and with renewed energy returned to regular walks with the children of the family. Although the cancer was terminal, Ebenezer and his family got to enjoy each other's company for a good year before he died.

HERBS AS MEDICINE

Our knowledge and use of plants as medicines began way back in history. Our ancestors observed animals and insects interact with plants and used them for healing. Through observation about the characteristics of a plant, speculation about its effects led to experimentation. Humans amassed knowledge about the benefits of plants and passed on to succeeding generations what we now consider herbal medicine. Plants are complementary partners with us. While we often take them for granted, survival wouldn't have been possible without them. They play a vital role in our food supply, shelter, clothing, fuel, and the air we breathe, and they are our medicines.

In today's world, where there is no shortage of therapeutic drugs, do herbal medicines have any significance? Indeed, herbal medicines alter body processes just as drugs do, and in many health problems, herbs can be as effective as and can be substituted for drugs.

Conventional medicine isolates a single active chemical component for therapeutic work. Herbalists would argue that the components of the entire plant work best when they stay together—that the synergy, or combined effect, of all the parts working together is greater than the parts working individually. Furthermore, combining herbs into a formula increases effectiveness.

Dosage is a factor important to drugs and herbs. Standardized doses for herbal medicines are typically presented as ranges: one to two teaspoons, one to four tablets, or one to six capsules, to be taken anywhere from one to four times a day. Such broad ranges are useful in finding the optimum combination that offers maximum benefits with the fewest side effects for the individual patient. It allows the herbalist to start prescriptions at the low end and gradually build up to the top of the recommended range. The body begins to accommodate the herbal preparation over a few days, and a watchful eye can be kept on the preparation's effects.

It is common for an herbalist to combine three or more herbal concentrates in a single formula. Such a combination is far safer than combining two or more therapeutic drugs. The risk of overdosing is almost nonexistent. Formulations give an herbalist the opportunity to add to the chief herbs one or two herbs to direct them to the organ that needs the treatment; other additions can slow down or speed up the action and effects, and the action is enhanced exponentially; and the herbalist can insert an herb that can mitigate possible side effects, such as a digestive problem.

Herbal medicines have strong selling points, so are they useful in cancer cases? In Chinese medicine (CM), cancer is looked at as a local manifestation of an underlying disease. A CM herbalist will focus on the whole body, the goal being to regulate body functions, maximize immunity, mitigate side effects of Western treatment, and enhance the effects of Western medicine (WM) treatment.

Cancer treatment as practiced in China and Europe integrates CM with WM and has been the mainstay of cancer treatment for decades. This type of treatment is an excellent adjunct to WM.[1] All the aspects of cancer—initiation, promotion, apoptosis, angiogenesis, and metastasis as well as prevention—are treated with herbal medicine.

When combined with conventional treatment, Chinese herbal medicine is effective in mitigating the side effects of anticancer agents and radiation, aids in recovering from surgery, and can adjust the body's systems (i.e., immune, nervous, digestive, and so on), shrink tumors, and improve quality of life. And CM herbs enhance long-term prognosis by as much as 50 percent.[2]

If surgery is indicated, herbs are used presurgery to prepare the patient. The choice of herbal ingredients depends on the findings of the herbalist when interviewing the owner and examining the patient. The plan would be to improve general health and, if needed, address the health of particular organs and systems. After surgery, herbs are the best approach to support digestive functions and promote recovery.

The trauma of surgery can suppress immune functions, allowing the escape of residual cancer cells from immune detection. The result can be recurrence and metastasis. Chinese herbal medicine restores all parts of the immune system, especially in the bone marrow.

Incorporating Chinese herbal medicine once chemotherapy or radiation begins improves long-term survival. Studies show that the use of Chinese herbal medicine with WM chemotherapy can affect metastasis rates dramatically. Gastric cancer survival rates were 3.2 years for patients having CM plus chemotherapy compared to 1.1 years for chemotherapy alone. Postsurgical lung cancer patients having CM with chemotherapy had a metastasis rate lower than patients with chemotherapy alone: 58.3 percent of postsurgical lung cancer patients having CM with chemotherapy had a metastasis rate lower than patients with chemotherapy alone, which was 12.5 percent. Studies on pancreatic cancer showed CM and chemotherapy survival rates of 16.3 months and, with chemotherapy alone, 7.5 months.[3]

The herbs used in cancer-combating formulas work on several fronts. They promote the rebuilding of red blood cells, decrease spleen weight and normalize liver functions, and improve appetite and promote weight gain. CM herbs prevent the body from losing ground to the effects of cancer. They offer the added benefit of being able to clean up the debris left behind by conventional treatment, revive energy levels, rebuild white blood cells, remove toxic loads, and heal tissue damaged by radiation. Overall, the addition of CM herbs creates a powerful impact.

Herb formulas used in China, Japan, and Europe are based on synergistic effects. To support the patient undergoing conventional treatment for cancer, a comprehensive approach to tumor eradication includes four elements: a formula consisting mostly of polysaccharides to help activate the immune system (more on this coming up) and then combined with antitoxin herbs, particularly those that contain alkaloid components for their antitumor properties; a mass-resolving mix of herbs since conventional treatment will eventually convert the malignancy into a mass of dead tissue; and an adjunct group to treat specific symptoms, such as fatigue or nausea.

The first three steps are followed throughout the cancer treatment phase. When the tumor is resolved, the immune-enhancing element is maintained for a period of several weeks to ensure the body's return to normalcy. Any adjunct therapies are used as needed during and after conventional treatment.

Herbs fit perfectly into any medical program because they are multifaceted and are varied. Roughly 80 percent of herbal material is from plants, shrubs, and trees. The other 20 percent comes from fungal material, minerals, and animal sources. The nonplant group is further subdivided into maritime material, such as shell, parts of sea animals and vegetables, and other animal sources, such as ancient bones.

Medicinal plants are rich in active ingredients, among them essential oils that can combat inflammation, infection, and pain. They contain an abundance of vitamins, especially A, E, and P, and minerals, such as calcium, magnetite, gypsum, and magnesium. They break down into highly complex sugar chains called polysaccharides. They also break down into amino acids. Herbs also supply organic acids, bile, and enzymes to facilitate digestion; alkaloids to resist infections and the growth of tumors; glucosides to boost the immune system; and tanins to inhibit discharges and act as antiseptics.

Science has been active in identifying which chemically active ingredients herb parts contain. Herbal profile analyses have verified why the seed, the stems, the leaves, the rhizome, or the roots are medically effective. New testing methods can also point out differences in quality among plants grown in different parts of the world and harvested at different times of the day and different seasons. Science has helped set benchmarks for the potency required in order for each herb to be effective.

In the process of preparing a treatment plan for cancer, several variables are considered. CM herbs are classified as mild, medium, or strong (not in potency but in effect) and would be prescribed according to which phase of treatment the patient is in. Strong herbs tend to act quickly and have almost immediate results. They are prescribed to treat severe and usually acute conditions that demand strong intervention. They are used sparingly and for a limited time. Medium-strength herbs are chosen primarily to stimulate chemical actions or calm chemical actions. Typically, they are prescribed either in higher potency for short-term use or in lower potency for long-term use. They can be given on an on-and-off basis. These herbs are generally used to support a pet through a long illness and in recuperation. Mild remedial herbs are usually restorative. These are put together from gentle herbs that work slowly, are cumulative in effect, and have no side effects; these can be used daily over long periods of time. Some of these herbs have a nutritive value and can even be considered medical foods. They are suitable for use in pets. Mild herbs are tonic herbs that extend life, slow down aging and degeneration in various organs, and heal.

How can you be sure that the CM herbs your pet is getting are safe? Safety depends on the raw materials themselves, where they are grown, and how they are processed. Many of the herbs in CM are typically grown and harvested in China and Taiwan. Herbal farms where acres of herbs are cultivated according to strict conditions for medical use are an important means of livelihood there.

The transforming of herbs into medicine is usually done in American companies. Plants are checked and cleaned, and the raw material is processed in traditional ways, such as being soaked in brine, mixed in honey, salted, charcoaled, or just plain dried. The herbs are ground into powders and can be purchased in that state by an herbalist; they are more likely to be made into capsules or tablets.

Tablets and capsules are convenient, but they're not the only form in which herbs are dispensed today. Dried herbs can be adapted into teas, baths, soaks, and poultices. Herbs also come in liquid extracts and tinctures that bypass the digestive process and are absorbed directly into the bloodstream.

American companies have become sophisticated in formulating herbs for use in cancer work; the formulas described in the following lists are extensively made in the United States and commonly used in cancer work. They come from the Seven Forests Company (see the "Resources" section in this book):

- *Chih-ko and Curcuma:* A formula designed to break down masses, tumors, solid cysts, and abscesses; it's typically used for solid tumors. It contains herbs to eliminate toxins and is most often taken along with another formula, such as one that can direct anticancer agents to the affected organ site. The formula is not suitable for blood cancers. It can be combined with the following for specific site cancers:
  - *Belancanda 15:* For lung tumors
  - *Blue Citrus:* For breast tumors
  - *Sparganium 12:* For gynecological tumors
  - *Laminaria 4, Prunella 8, or Scrophularia 12:* For soft tumors
  - *Eupolyphaga tablets:* For abdominal masses
  - *Zedoaria tablets:* For hard tumors
  - *Oxymartrine:* Not for tumors but to prevent leukopenia, or a decrease in the number of white blood cells, during therapy

In addition to these formulas, there are several that help keep the body as normal as possible during WM treatment:

- *Cordyceps 9:* Traditionally given to a patient in deteriorating health due to a chronic disease and can be used to help patients detoxify from steroid medications and other anti-inflammatory drugs.
- *Ganoderma 18:* For patients who suffer from weakness and deteriorating changes in organ systems. These changes can arise from the impact of a serious illness or from the side effects of toxic drug therapies.
- *Antler 8:* A formula taken with *Ganoderma* to reverse bone marrow suppression and red blood cell problems.
- *Ginseng 18:* Good choice for dealing with indigestion, diarrhea, bloating, and poor nutritional status that often accompanies and/or follows WM treatment.

- *Gynostemma tablets:* Will complement WM treatment and is best given before medical therapies begin to boost immune functions. It should be continued for a minimum of four to six weeks after any intensive medical therapies are ended.
- *Coricepium:* Can be added to *Gynostemma* to increase levels of polysaccharides.
- *Quercenol:* Can be added for an antioxidant effect.
- *Astragalus 10:* Restores deficiencies in the immune system. This formula should be taken in substantial amounts for initial therapy and, after improvement, maintained at a lower dosage. In China, Astragalus is often the cornerstone of integrative oncology.
- *Otolith tablets:* Can be used paired with WM treatment for brain cancer. It treats convulsions, tremors, and swellings.
- *Reconciling tablets:* Treats inflammation and tissue damage.
- *Recovery pills:* Used mostly for postsurgical therapy and treats pain, weakness, loss of mobility, and impaired circulation while reversing damage to tissue.
- *Dan Shen Pian:* Helps reduce fibrosis.

All of the above herb formulas have the major advantage of low to no toxicity; they can be used long term without ill effects. Patients who have food allergies or digestive problems or who seem highly sensitive should be started at a reduced dose and slowly increased to a higher dose.

The normal dosage of Chinese herbs in pill or powder form is at least 0.5 to 1 gram per day for small dogs and cats and 1 to 1.5 grams for a large dog. Give herbs and drugs at least two hours apart. Whenever possible, give on an empty stomach; however, capsules can be opened and tablets ground into powder and added to food if it proves difficult to pill the animal. Birds can be treated by sprinkling pinches of powdered herbs onto food sources, such as vegetables.

HERBS: POWERFUL ALLIES IN CANCER TREATMENT

Polysaccharides appear to be the common denominator in many of the herbs in cancer formulas. They are found throughout the plant kingdom, and the idea that polysaccharides might inhibit tumor growth by enhancing immune functions was first presented in 1958. Unlike commonly used

WM cancer drugs, they have no cytotoxic effect and are nontoxic. Instead, they help eliminate tumors by promoting immune system attack against malignant cells. In Japanese research studies, implanted sarcomas were treated with either a neutral solution or one of the polysaccharides of the medicinal mushroom subset of natural anticancer agents. The National Cancer Center in Japan reported that complete tumor elimination was experienced in about 80 percent of cancer-induced animals. It's reported that the mushroom used—*Maitake* D-Fraction—shows strong anticancer activity by increasing the tumor-killing ability of natural killer cells and enhances other immune cells' production of interleukin-1.[4]

Korean researchers tested an extract of the polysaccharides from the *Ganoderma* mushroom against implanted tumor cells. In the control group, after 28 days, the average tumor weight was 4.5 grams, but in mice receiving the extract, it was only 0.6 grams. A third of the mice receiving *Ganoderma* had a complete remission of the cancer, but none of the control mice experienced complete remission.[5] What medicinal mushroom studies showed was that in certain strains of mice, some polysaccharides demonstrated effective antitumor activity while others did not. The research pointed out that there are main differences among strains of mice in their cell surface receptors and that the polysaccharides were interacting with a limited set of these receptors. One strain of mice would benefit, and another would not. This breakthrough gave researchers the idea of using a mixture of polysaccharides, in these cases mushroom polysaccharides, rather than a single one. A combination of six to nine medicinal mushrooms is now used in cancer treatment. Polysaccharides from other natural sources are also combined for their synergistic properties. The dosage consumed and the duration of their consumption are important. When mice are fed polysaccharides at 10, 20, or 30 percent of their diets, the antitumor activity increased in direct correlation with the dosage.

Plants with alkaloids as chief active ingredients are another group of herbs extensively researched for their potential anticancer effects. Alkaloids were the earliest major drugs obtained from plants. Morphine, quinine, caffeine, strychnine, atropine, and ephedrine are some examples of drugs with alkaloid isolates from plants. Chinese medicinal use of these agents is to promote phagocytosis, or the inhibition of tumor cells. The anticancer drugs vincristine and vinblastine was developed from alkaloids in plants that have been used in cancer treatment for decades.

HERBS AND VIRUSES

Modern medicine is slowly beginning to discover the hidden role of some viruses and bacteria in cancer initiation and development. Viruses act as both initiators and promoters, silently invading and contributing to more than a dozen malignancies. The cancer toll from pathogens such as viruses and bacteria may turn out to be higher than ever thought. The hepatitis B and C viruses, which attack the liver, take over healthy cells and cause inflammation that damages the organ. In humans, about 10 percent of patients who suffer chronic hepatitis stand an increased chance of developing cancer.

Viruses are virulent and prey on a body already suffering from another disease. Some, such as those in the herpes family, are opportunistic, waiting for the immune system to collapse and then invading and causing problems. There are rapidly transforming viruses and slowly transforming ones, depending on the genetics of the host, the presence of trauma, immunosuppression status, hormone cofactors, and chemical carcinogens. They can have a double-punch effect: an acute stage and a later chronic stage. It may take many years for the cells' genomes carrying the virus to activate (chicken pox in childhood and shingles later). They have been thought to initiate cancer. Retrovirus material has been detected in the RNA of lymphoma cancer cells. The papilloma virus is associated with laryngeal, cervical, and squamous cell carcinoma.

The herpes virus is an example of a slow, latent virus; it can be acute, chronic, and recurrent. More than 25 different strains make up the herpes family, and humans and animals alike are natural hosts. Herpes is suspected to be involved in cancer. These retroviruses are believed to lead to cancers such as leukemia. The Epstein-Barr virus has been associated with nasopharyngeal carcinoma, Hodgkin's disease, and some lymphomas.

If your pet has a viral condition, he needs to be treated with agents that kill off much of the viral material and bring down what is called the "viral load." Chinese herbal medicine has some answers:

- *Coptis:* For cholera, anthrax, intestinal infections, and Newcastle virus
- *Scute:* For adenovirus, rhinovirus, and feline immunodeficiency virus (FIV)
- *Isatis:* For FIV, encephalitis, viral skin conditions, and influenza
- *Phelldendron:* For intestinal viruses

A large number of formulas are also available. The following are from Health Concerns:

- *Artestatin:* Treats acute infections; used in conjunction with conventional therapy for cryptosporidiosis and shigella
- *Astra C:* For the prevention of viral flu
- *Astra Isatis:* For chronic viral infection such as chronic fatigue syndrome, herpes simplex, and hepatitis
- *Clear Heat:* For viral, bacterial, and fungal infections; chronic viral warts; and chronic herpes
- *Astras Isatis, Power Mushrooms, Enhance, or Cordyceps:* For chronic immune dysfunction syndrome (CIDS) and chronic fatigue syndrome (CFS)
- *Coptis Purge Fire:* For acute situations and intense, localized, and inflamed outbreaks
- *Ecliptex:* For hepatitis
- *Enhance:* Used for immune enhancement and to treat chronic viral inflammation and infection as in chronic fatigue immune dysfunction syndrome (CFIDS), CFS, and herpes
- *Hepatoplex One:* For hepatitis C
- *Phellostatin:* Antibacterial, antifungal, and antiviral systemic conditions

The following are from the Seven Forests Company:

- *Bidens:* For viral and bacterial infections including hepatitis and cytomegalovirus (CMV)
- *Bupleurum and Gardenia:* For hepatitis and difficult-to-kill infections
- *Isatis 6:* For any viral infection
- *Paris 7:* For chronic viral infections
- *Red Peony:* For herpes zoster
- *Salvia/Ligustrum:* For hepatitis B and C
- *Viola 12:* For fever of an unknown origin and lymph node swelling of unknown origin

The following are from White Tiger:

- *Baicalcumin:* For viral hepatitis, lung viruses, and inhibition of DNA activation of chronic viruses

- *Myrolea-B:* For viral infections, such as flu and coxsackie, and bacterial infections, such as strep and leptospirosis

POINTS TO KEEP IN MIND

Herbal medicine is not a hit-or-miss therapy. It is grounded in science and has been clinically used for centuries and guaranteed from research and use in China, Japan, and Europe to be a big help for a pet with cancer. You need to develop a plan that utilizes the best results for your pet's individual needs. You need an herbalist to help you. The integration of traditional Chinese herbal medicine and modern CM with WM in cancer treatment needs to be in skilled and knowledgeable hands. The focus of WM treatment is on the cancer itself and can reduce the cancer load. CM offers supportive treatment on multiple levels: enabling the patient to get through the WM treatment, coming out of it in the best possible physical condition with maximum survival time, and providing the lowest possible chance of metastasis.

Costs of integrating CM and WM run from a few cents to five dollars a day, depending on what herbal ingredients are used. Herbal preparations have long shelf lives. An unopened bottle stored at room temperature retains 95 percent of its active ingredients for up to six months after the expiration date. Dried herbs should be stored in tightly closed glass containers and kept in a cool, dark place. Capsules and tablets need only be kept dry. To prevent spoilage, oil-based salves must be refrigerated on opening.

A general rule for dosing is the following:

Small dogs and cats: 1 capsule or tablet twice a day; if liquid form, 8 to 10 drops twice a day
Medium-size dogs: 2 capsules or tablets twice a day; if liquid, 15 to 20 drops twice a day
Large dogs: 2 to 3 capsules or tablets twice a day; if liquid, 20 to 30 drops a day
Birds: 1 capsule or tablet crushed into powder and sprinkled on various foods; if liquid, 5 to 10 drops into the water and/or on food

A program of prevention can begin in midlife with off-and-on herbal therapy three or four times a year. The frequency doubles with every two-year interval; for example, a dog at six or seven years of age would have an herbal regime every three or four months, depending on his size, and a dog of eight or nine would have an herbal regime every two months. Size is considered because large- and giant-breed dogs need to be started much earlier, at age three or four, and a small or toy breed can be started later, at six or seven. If the pet has a genetic predisposition to cancer initiation, such as the currently popular breeds of the Golden retriever, Labrador retriever, and Bernese mountain dog, prevention needs to be continuous from early on and more aggressive as the dog grows older.

You don't need to transform your kitchen into an apothecary to employ herbs in your life. Don't run out and buy all sorts of equipment and ingredients; you need only a few well-chosen herbal extracts or tinctures on hand for everyday use and one or two machines. To take maximum advantage of the benefits of herbs, you may want to buy a juicer, with which you can extract the nutrients from the fruits and vegetables used as a base for herbal drinks and soups. A blender will allow you to puree ingredients with herbs, and a food processor is a great way to mix everything together and prevent the pet from picking out only what he likes.

In China, herbal medicine and acupuncture have been a large part of oncology treatment for over 50 years. It is routine to use both WM and CM together, making a comprehensive plan for cancer patients whose goal is to improve treatment outcome, quality of life, and survival.[6] Your pet can benefit from what has been learned to improve the outcome of treatment and survival. See Appendix D.

14

THE WONDERS OF
THE IMMUNE SYSTEM

In many ways, the immune system is the most magnificent system in the body; it rivals the brain in terms of complexity, subtlety, and self-awareness. Yet it can be the most ignored system in day-to-day living. Indeed, it typically works so well that we and the people we depend on for medical care tend to forget about it. In many ways, we even seem to do everything in our power to destroy it. For example, just one can of soda will depress the immune system by 50 percent for six hours. We and our pets can't be in good health, nor can we eliminate a disease, unless our immune systems are working at optimum efficiency. Without an immune system, we and our pets would quickly fall prey to almost every bacteria, virus, and parasite in our world. Our "self" could not protect itself from "nonself," and the body would age at an alarming speed.

Have you ever wondered what your pet's immune system does all day? If you thought about it, you would probably guess that it must work hard, but does it get tired or worn out, like other parts of the body? Does it require medical care like a heart or a liver? If it breaks down, how can it be fixed? Why does one pet become ill when another doesn't? Three healthy people can breathe the same germs at the same moment: one may develop pneumonia, another a cold, and the third nothing. This suggests that susceptibility is individual. Evidence suggests that germs don't simply jump into us and cause disease. A germ does indeed challenge the body, but the end result is entirely dependent on the body's ability to resist through its defense system.

The prime role of an immune system is protection. It does its job by being a complex organization, delegating responsibility to its many parts, much as giant megacorporations do. It functions through two separate but interconnected branches: humoral immunity and cell-mediated, or cellular, immunity. The humoral part relies greatly on blood-borne factors: the types of blood cells and their subgroups and the antibodies the blood cells produce. Cellular immunity does not depend on antibody response; it recognizes intruders directly. Both types provide constant surveillance. They can quickly respond to foreign organisms and mount a campaign of destruction using specialized cells, or they can neutralize their disease-causing effects by eliminating their toxins.

The system stands guard over the cells in the body, ensuring that they do not become abnormal. The immune system has the capacity not only to identify every single cell in the body but also to recognize it as "friendly" or "foreign," belonging or not belonging. When it identifies a foreign invader, it quickly develops a customized defense weapon to target the intruder's weak spot. Next, it rapidly reproduces the weapons it needs in massive quantities to crush the intruder. Once the threat is eliminated, the system has the awareness to shut itself off.

As wonderful as this level of protection is, there is yet another amazing aspect of the immune system: its intelligence. Once it has defeated an invader, the immune system remembers that invader and the defenses it used to defeat it. If it should meet the invader again, even years later, it will mount the appropriate defense instantly. Furthermore, it is so sophisticated that it can identify a cell that is "going over to the enemy," as it were. Out of all the trillions of cells in the body, the immune system can tell which one single cell has mutated and become abnormal, even cancerous. In most cases, it is able to destroy it before it can do harm. And it does this thousands of times a day. In addition, this remarkable system has the ability to communicate with each and every part of itself.

Obviously, the system has to have all its parts in good working order to function at all these levels. All the parts begin in the blood cells, both red and white, which begin their lives as stem cells in the bone marrow. At some point, these undifferentiated stem cells begin to develop into red, or oxygen-bearing, cells, or the white cells of the immune system with their individual characteristics. Those that are white become leukocytes; these will further differentiate into four main types: lymphocytes, phagocytes, granulocytes, and dendritic cells.

Lymphocytes are the key operatives of the entire system, numbering about 1 trillion in a healthy body. They also divide into three main classes: B-cells, T-cells, and natural killer (NK) cells. Each B-cell is programmed to make one specific antibody to defend itself against one specific invader. For example, one B-cell produces an antibody to defend the body against only one particular strain of flu, while another B-cell produces the antibody for a different strain of flu. (An antibody is a protein capable of binding to and destroying or neutralizing one specific foreign substance called an antigen.)

The T-cells are even smarter. Not only do they know the difference between cells of the body and invading cells, but they are also able to distinguish between normal, healthy cells and mutated, rogue cells. T-cells carry markers on their surface. They all have a T-3 marker identification; some also carry a T-4 marker, which makes them "helper" cells. These help activate many of the different subtypes of cells in the system. And some carry a T-8 marker, making them capable of identifying rogue, mutated cells and cells invaded by a virus. This subgroup is also known as the cytotoxic T-cells, or "suppressor cells," and they have a big killer instinct, attacking and disintegrating cells that have been infected or that are malignant.

Whenever B- or T-cells become activated, some will end up as memory cells. They encode a "memory" of the specific antigen associated with the invader; if there is a next time, the system will respond without delay.

The NK cells attack a whole range of microbes; they are nondiscriminating. In addition, they particularly like to go after tumor cells. They kill on contact through lethal blasts of potent chemicals that can burn holes in target cells, causing them to leak, burst open, and die.

The phagocytes are large, white cells that eat and digest pathogens. The group consists of monocytes, neutrophils, and macrophages. Monocytes migrate to the site of an invasion when needed and, once stimulated, become macrophages. The macrophages are thought to play a primary role in anticancer immunity. Stimulation of macrophage activity has been associated with decreased tumor growth as well as decreased tumor incidence. Their key role is as scavengers eating up worn-out cells and other wastes in the body. Of interest to researchers is the fact that macrophages play a key role in fasting. When you put a pet on a fast, he is not creating new waste in the body; one of the benefits of a fast is giving the macrophages a chance to get ahead of the game in terms of cleaning out longstanding debris.

Granulocytes include eosinophils, basophils, neutrophils, and mast cells. Eosinophils like to eat parasites, neutrophils enjoy bacteria and dead matter, and basophils go to work in allergic responses. Dendritic cells, with long, threadlike tentacles, wrap up used, impotent lymphocytes and carry them off for removal.

Organs play key roles in immune response; therefore, removal of an organ such as the spleen may seriously compromise the immune system. The major players are the bone marrow, which produces the cells of the system; the thymus, which trains the T-cells; the lymph nodes, whose role it is to transport the cells throughout the body; the spleen, which serves as a staging area and a blood filtration plant; the tonsils; the adenoids; and the appendix. Each one is important and irreplaceable.

There is also a complementary immune system—a secondary system that kicks in when the immune system is totally overwhelmed. It consists of approximately 25 proteins/enzymes that activate in a cascading sequence and end with what's called the "membrane attack complex." The name describes the action; the complex attacks the cell walls—the membranes— of the invaders. This system can also help get rid of "circulating immune complexes," proteins that are not digested in the intestines and leak out into the bloodstream, looking, for all intents and purposes, like "foreigners." These complexes provoke attack and, in large numbers, will initiate an allergic reaction. They also accumulate in the body's soft tissues, giving rise to inflammation and becoming instigators of an autoimmune problem.

We've now seen how the immune system works—how it identifies invaders and mounts a response—but how does it communicate with itself? The answer is through powerful messengers secreted by cells called cytokines. Among them are some you have probably heard of, such as interferon, interleukins, and tumor necrosis factor. Billions of these tiny messengers carry out various intelligent checks and balances throughout the immune system—guiding it, regulating it, marshaling it, and resting it.

With all these resources, you would think the system would be invulnerable. Not true. There are many problems that can and do occur. The immune system can be overwhelmed by too many invaders. This is very common in natural disasters; rescuers saw this in dogs left behind in the wake of Hurricane Katrina and in the search-and-rescue dogs of 9/11. Or the immune system becomes weakened and vulnerable. An animal with a recurrent or chronic infection will live in a cycle of repeated infection, damage, and subsequently lowered resistance. The system can become misprogrammed and lose its ability to identify invaders or mutated cells. And the system can become misprogrammed in another way, mistakenly identifying healthy cells as the enemy and beginning to attack and destroy itself. And, of course, there are animals (and humans) who are born missing some key component.

As wonderful as the immune system is, it doesn't always recognize cancer as the potential threat it is: cancer cells can look so similar to normal cells that they go unregistered as dangerous. Cancer cells, like viruses and other pathogens and parasites, are always finding ways to sidestep recognition, adjusting their disguises to make them indistinguishable from normal cells. Even when recognized as dangerous, cancer cells are not necessarily vulnerable to destruction. Your pet could have a type of cancer resistant to immune responses and various treatment protocols.

Fortunately, the immune system has many parts, and each part can be enhanced and brought into an overall treatment strategy. Since the purpose of the body's immune system is to defend against attack and initiate repair, the better it does that, the healthier the body. To help this process, we need to address the key areas we've identified. We have to improve overall immune function, that is, optimize it with a multifaceted plan. And we need to give the system help in its targeting of all pathogens. We can do this. It is within our means to improve the functioning of the immune system, and we don't need to use expensive measures. We can adopt an approach of utilizing natural agents, which are far safer than drugs with far fewer side effects and which provide an impact as powerful as any of their pharmaceutical counterparts.

WHAT YOU CAN DO TO BOOST
THE SYSTEM'S POWER

If your pet is undergoing conventional cancer treatment, you can help to maximize his immune system in order to reduce the risk of complications. A significant drop in his white blood cell count can put your pet at risk of developing a serious infection. If he has undergone conventional chemotherapy, it makes sense to give him infection-fighting, herbal formulas, especially if he is to be put in day care or doggie group activities. The immune cells most involved in destroying invading pathogens are the neutrophils. If symptoms such as coughing, diarrhea, fever, chills and shaking, earache, or other acute problems develop, you need to take steps to get the neutrophil numbers up.

For the common cold or influenza, use Yin Qiao Jie Du Pian (Pine Mountain brand). This formula is a popular remedy in tablet form for early-stage influenza and the common cold. Use it at high dosage at the first sign of a viral infection; this can potentially halt further development of the illness, even before a full symptom picture appears. Propol-Gold (White Tiger brand) is a small formula aimed at bacterial, fungal, and viral infections in the intestines, along with gum and oral infections and sinus infections.

Then avoid giving raw foods that could contain pathogens and parasites. This means meats, along with fruits and vegetables. Cook well-washed fruits and vegetables as well as meat or poultry. Keep the litter box scrupulously clean. Keep your pet confined and keep contact with other animals (or even children or adults who have recently been vaccinated) to a minimum. Don't walk a dog where he may be cut, scraped, or bruised. Keep him from scratching himself inordinately. Wash your hands before petting or cleaning your animal, and allow your pet to get plenty of rest.

This is the time to supply your pet with the best nutritional foods and supplements. Reduce dietary saturated fats but increase omega-3 fatty acids. Include vitamin E with the omega-3; the vitamin will counteract any problems, such as rancidity and NK cell depression. Reduce iron intake, which means avoid serving red meat; a vegetable-rich diet will keep iron levels in check. Feed him whole grains, legumes, fruits, and vegetables—especially carotene-rich ones—and fish, such as salmon, to achieve a higher ratio of T-helper cells to T-suppressor cells. A new ratio is desirable for eliminating any cancer cells that remain after chemotherapy. In addition, this diet increases the activity of NK cells. Give him a food-based multivitamin. Most patients will be deficient in these vital nutrients after a chemotherapy treatment. Vitamin C, for example, improves the activity of NK cells and overall T-cell functions. Zinc and selenium increase NK activity, along with neutrophil and macrophage phagocytosis. Make one of the elixirs or drinks suggested in Appendix B, such as the high-mineral drink for daily use.

Introducing antioxidants into your dog's life supports the active functioning of the immune system. One of the most powerful antioxidants is glutathione. It is an amino acid and a key component of all lymphocytes; all lymphocytes require sufficient levels of intracellular glutathione to work properly. A good, full spectrum of antioxidants boosts the immune system in multiple ways. Nutrients from organically grown fruits and vegetables—the cruciferous family, citrus fruit, soy, legumes, bright-colored foods (e.g., carrots, squash, and berries), and deep-colored foods (e.g., kale, cabbage, and Brussels sprouts)—block carcinogen activity, increase carcinogen detoxification, block the action of tumor promoters, scavenge free radicals that cause fast aging, force rogue cells to commit suicide, cut off blood circulation to tumor cells, and keep inflammation minimized.

If there are no complications or acute or adverse reactions, plan on supplying your pet with terrain modifiers. A multiagent approach would include glutathione, bromelain, and quercetin enzymes in a mixture of other enzymes. These reduce metastatic potential and increase cell membrane permeability, allowing more of the chemotherapy drugs to be carried through to the cell's interior. The enzymes can also inhibit the development of drug resistance. Add an *Astragalus* formula, perhaps Astragalus 10+ (Seven Forests brand) or Astra 8 or a *Ganoderma*-based formula, such as Ganoderma 18 (Seven Forests brand) to restore immune function or Composition A (Seven Forests brand), which is required for optimal activation of T-lymphocytes and the prevention of leukopenia (low white blood cell count). This last formula contains *Astragalus* and *Ganoderma* herbs as well as antitoxin herbs, such as *Andrographis*.

And use acupuncture absolutely. Used immediately after chemotherapy, this therapy influences leukocyte counts dramatically. It works well on radiation-induced edema, reduces nausea and vomiting, and, in general, results in improvement in approximately 95 percent of patients.

Lactoferrin is a cytokine found in the most vulnerable-to-attack parts of the body, such as the gut and the urinary tract. Lactoferrin inhibits virus replication, including the herpes viruses. It inhibits tumor growth and metastasis; it is directly toxic to both bacteria and yeast and helps prevent their overgrowth in the gut. It activates neutrophil cells (the killers and cleaners of the system). Stimulating lactoferrin production in the body and maintaining healthy levels of this protection is the work of the intestinal flora, or probiotics.

Introducing essential fatty acids into the plan helps to keep the immune system properly programmed so it doesn't attack itself. Cleaning out the liver with an effective, flush-and-rebuild program improves the liver's ability to produce immune factors. Cleaning out the blood with herbal cleansers and balancing the pH of the blood are two other key elements in improving immune function. Regular exercise is a definite optimizer. And, of course, we must bolster immune surveillance by means of the best food possible. The message is simple, and the message is lifesaving. Solutions are definitely within your grasp.

Above all, keep constant your appreciation of your animal. My client Cheryl discovered a great deal about herself and her dog, Deja vue, when the dog became ill. Deja had been with Cheryl through an unhappy relationship that ended in her becoming a single mother of a baby boy. Cheryl explained that this dog was very special. When she noticed a very small lump developing on Deja's leg in a very short span of time, she became alarmed. Deja was diagnosed with a ligament problem and put on a program of medication, but there was no change in the growth of the lump or her inability to use the leg. Cheryl switched to another veterinarian who, after a series of X-rays, diagnosed cancer in one of her long leg bones. The veterinarian recommended surgical removal. If the leg were left untreated, it would continue to cause a great deal of pain; eventually the bone would be destroyed enough to fracture. The surgery would eliminate the primary tumor and offer a reprieve for a short time from metastasis.

Deja handled the surgery well and adjusted to her new gait. Chemotherapy was suggested, which Cheryl decided against, yet she was not able to stop thinking about her dog's future and the possibility of the cancer showing up somewhere else in the dog's body. She decided to pursue an unconventional approach.

Cheryl, Deja, and I began working together about two months after the surgery. Deja had acupuncture therapy once a week for a month, then once every four to six weeks after that. Cheryl gave the dog doses of herbal medicine and a great, high-nutrition diet. Since osteosarcoma in dogs is likely to spread to the lungs, Cheryl made sure that X-rays were done periodically. Deja got through a year with no signs of ill health. Well into the second year, however, Deja started coughing. An ultrasound at that time showed signs of tumor growth and lungs full of fluid. The lungs were drained to make her comfortable, and we started a wait-and-see period. Deja started to lose her appetite and energy; when she refused to go for walks, Cheryl made the decision to euthanize her.

When dogs with osteosarcoma are treated with surgery alone, the survival rate is about 100 days for 90 percent of dogs. Surgical treatment is usually considered palliative. When chemotherapy is added, survival increases to 180 to 400 days for 50 percent of dogs. Deja outlived the statistics. With acupuncture and herbal medicine, Deja lived longer than the maximum expectations for animals receiving these conventional treatments. Cheryl was spared expensive and toxic interventions, and she was given the gift of one and a half more years with her dog. Meanwhile, Deja vue had a good quality of life until the end.

15

NEVER GIVE UP

The longer we and our pets live, the more rapidly our potential for acquiring cancer-inducing genetic mutations accelerates. This is due to the chromosomes that house genes; they become fragile, and the molecular repair kits that keep the molecule ends covered and protected with protein decay. This decaying process is especially prevalent in cells that divide a great deal, such as the cells that line the ducts of the breast and prostate, the air passages of the lungs, and the intestines.

The process of mutative change can be either gradual or cataclysmic. If a particularly traumatic event occurs, chromosomes fracture suddenly, and the broken pieces randomly fuse and copy themselves. At sites where chromosomes are mashed together, genes critical to growth regulation may be deleted, mutated, or increased.

To become cancerous, genes must have particular proteins that actively induce cancer. These genes are called oncogenes, and their proteins are constantly demanding cell division. Just as bad as mutating and replicating itself faster and faster, a cell can lose its tumor-suppressor genes. As the name signifies, its proteins detect important mutations; when they find DNA in bad shape, they signal the cell to commit suicide. In aging cells, there are more possibilities for oncogenes and fewer and fewer tumor-suppressor genes. When damage is done, the cell adapts until it has only one function: dividing and surviving in its new form. It is now a full-blown cancer cell. It has created a specialized organ within an organ. It steals its own supporting cells and its own blood supply from the host.

Most cancers are detected after a tumor has been growing and active for some time. This is the point at which conventional therapies step in, and some combination of surgery, chemotherapy, radiation, or other therapy is employed to reduce or eliminate the tumor. This is cytoreduction (cyto = cell). An effective cytoreduction phase brings either partial remission or a complete remission. In a partial remission, evidence of cancer is still visible on examination. In a complete remission, there seems to be no visible cancer; however, residual cancer cells may be there but invisible.

Eliminating primary tumors may have no impact on micrometastases: the cells that may have escaped and set themselves up in the blood, lymph nodes, or distant organs. These cells have undergone genetic makeovers that leave them resistant to treatment and harder to kill. Months or years later, they will reappear. Since it's impossible to know whether residual cells will remain quiet or come back stronger than ever, requiring yet more toxic, aggressive therapies, you can sit back and adopt a wait-and-see attitude, or you can come as close as possible to eliminating the disease by attacking it with natural, integrative therapies.

The goal is to keep tumor growth nonexistent as long as possible. We can all live with malignant cells in our bodies as long as they don't begin multiplying and metastasizing. Whether residual tumor cells are visible or not, this is the time to hold on to any gains made during the conventional therapy. Even cancers that have resisted conventional treatments can be contained enough for the patient to live with cancer as a chronic disease. Therefore, while any statement made that a cancer is in remission should be viewed optimistically, resistant cells often remain, and the patient needs a long-term program that fights regrowth. The longer your pet is in remission, the better the chances of beating the disease. From this point on, your pet's life is never going to be the same as it once was. His life has to be different now for as long as he lives.

Baby was diagnosed with cancer in the oviduct. The small bird started showing signs of ill health, and, after X-rays and a biopsy, she was diagnosed and given a three-month prognosis. Working with me, her human companion began a program of herbal medicine. Baby was fed a liquid, herbal mix with a syringe three times a day, and dry herbs were sprinkled on her food. Baby beat the odds by living for two more years.

The fact is that when your pet's conventional treatment is over, you are virtually on your own. Conventional care has no real follow-up plan beyond monitoring; you can hope for the best outcome or wait for the next chapter. But there is a much better way to go forward.

If your pet is in a containing phase with the presence of a visible tumor, he needs rehabilitation. Some patients I've seen have been greatly weakened due to the severity of the cancer and other preexisting medical problems. Some end up debilitated by the toxicity of chemotherapy. Whatever the condition, this is where we begin. A rehabilitation program has several parts. If your pet now has a damaged digestive system, he may be weak, not taking in enough calories, and, as a consequence, wasting away.

Cook some peppermint tea or some slices of ginger and replace his plain water with one of these. These primarily stimulate the appetite. Look up the "bitters" recipe in appendix C and try using that. If your pet is chronically nauseous, give him a digestive enzyme mix a few minutes before he is offered food. The homeopathic remedies Nux Vomica and Carbo Vegetabilis are a wonderful duo for upset stomach and work rapidly. Definitely offer him a hearty, easy-to-digest meal. Also consider the Chinese formula Atractylodes tablets (Seven Forests brand) for intestinal disorders, such as cramps, aching, and diarrhea.

If your pet has trouble swallowing because of an inflamed throat, try slippery elm. An amino acid mix with extra glutamine is good to overcome muscle loss. The amino acid glutamine should always be considered if there are digestive problems. Omega-3 EFA, 1 to 2 grams a day, will inhibit the production of inflammatory agents. (Inflammation secreted by tumors plays a major role in poor health or cachexia [wasting] due to cancer.) Vitamins C and E reduce some inflammatory agents as well. If fever is a problem, particularly idiopathic type, or if the fever is of an unknown origin, the Chinese medicine formula Rhemannia 6 (Liu Wei Di Huang Wan) is a great answer. If the pet develops anemia, the formula Tang-Kuei tablets (Seven Forests brand) will build up the blood and get it circulating.

REMISSION IS ONLY THE BEGINNING

Being told that your pet is in remission is no reason to slacken off. Remission does not equate with cure. A body is cured of cancer if the tumor was caught very early (and I stress the word "very") and was removed by surgery with clean margins. It is in these types of cases that the patient has the best chance of not harboring malignant cells somewhere else in the body. But most cases need ongoing, comprehensive care, and you need to be proactive in instituting a remission maintenance plan. That certainly includes monitoring your pet's status with lab tests and imaging for a recurrence in the year or two after treatment since early detection allows for a better prognosis and therapy that's less invasive.

Cancer patients are also at a higher risk of developing a second cancer, an entirely new disease, years after treatment. This type of cancer reflects the pet's terrain being hospitable to growing malignancies. The cause of the first cancer may be the cause of the second cancer, or the second cancer may have been initiated as a result of treatment. Whatever the cause, reducing the risk has to be your priority.

If your pet's oncologist tells you that there is nothing more he can do for your pet, it means there is nothing in his conventional medical kit that can help. That leaves the kind of medicine written about in this book as the default therapy. I'll be the first to admit that some of the natural agents recommended here have not had a long history of tests and clinical trials. However, they are well known and well regarded in other parts of the world—namely, Europe, China, and Japan. Some have been used for decades in cancer treatment. Let's go through the choices.

Modulating inflammation is an important part of integrative cancer therapy. Let's examine the link between inflammation and cancer initiation, promotion, progression, angiogenesis (the development of new blood vessels, in this case to feed tumor growth), and metastasis. In many cancers, there is a relationship between cancer pathology and particular inflammatory agents, among them prostaglandins and leukotrienes. (This connection has been looked at as far back as the 1970s.) Agents that inhibit the enzymes that synthesize prostaglandins and leukotrienes—called COX and LOX—are useful in controlling cancer. COX has been documented in the malignant tissues of cancer patients and correlates with tumor size, stage, recurrence rates, metastasis, and patient survival. LOX is generated by many cancers and plays a significant role in promoting the proliferation and spread of cancer. Newer research proposes a role for anti-inflammatory agents in the prevention of colon, pancreatic, breast, prostate, lung, skin, urinary, bladder, and liver cancers. These agents, plus other nontoxic, anti-inflammatory strategies, may provide a big part of the solution to the challenges of both prevention and therapy.[1]

Dietary intake of fats is a primary consideration; the total concentration of fatty acids in cell membranes determines whether inflammation will occur. The right diet will reduce available nutrients (arachidonic acid) for the production of prostaglandins and leukotrienes while increasing the availability of anti-inflammatory compounds. Cancer cells have greatly increased amounts of arachidonic acid; animal fats and omega-6 vegetable oils increase the acid content. Dietary sources of arachidonic acid can be minimized through the restriction of red meats, dairy products, and eggs. However, once your pet has adapted to a plant-rich, mostly vegetarian, whole-foods diet, you may add in moderation lean red meat; nonfat, organic dairy products; skinless, free-range poultry; and omega-3-rich eggs. Refined and processed vegetable oils should be completely eliminated from the diet and replaced with organically processed, cold-pressed olive oil. Any omega-6 should come from whole foods and only in limited amounts. Meanwhile, dietary sources of omega-3 can be markedly increased, especially in the form of cold-water fish. And, in general, your pet's diet should contain lots of antioxidant-rich food: deeply pigmented vegetables and fruits. High inflammation levels are known to deplete the body's antioxidant stores. Taking care to replace these antioxidants in cancer patients increases the body's reserves. Antioxidants can decrease COX levels as well.

But don't stop there; add phytonutrients to further modulate the inflammatory process. A large number of natural compounds offer anti-inflammatory effects. Among these are the enzymes bromelain and quercetin and herbs such as boswellia, curcumin, devil's claw, milk thistle, *picrorrhiza*, *scutellaria*, and bilberry. Using multiple natural agents yields synergistic effects, addressing both COX and LOX inhibition. Fish oil supplements supplant arachidonic acid in cell membranes, limiting the production of prostaglandins and leukotrienes. Studies in human brain cancer showed favorable results on metastatic brain lesions using moderate doses of fish oil and the flavonoid silymarin, an active ingredient in the herb milk thistle. The combination resulted in an increase in survival duration of 64 percent compared to unsupplemented patients.[2]

What will result if we put into effect a plan like this? First, fish oil supplements will inhibit the making of arachidonic acid, thus decreasing the possibility of COX and LOX by-product formation. Add bromelain, and you interfere with the growth of malignant cells. Use curcumin, and you induce apoptosis (cell death) while inhibiting angiogenesis. This plant has also been shown to enhance NK-cell-mediated tumor remission. The traditional Chinese medicine formula *Chih-ko* and *Curcuma* (Seven Forests brand) is an example of a centuries-old combination of herbs used to treat hard and soft tumor types, not blood cancers. It is most often combined with other formulas, according to the specific cancer involved. The traditional Chinese medicine formula *Picrorrhiza* 11 (Seven Forests brand) can be used with it, as it is designed for treating a wide range of infections and inflammatory conditions. And either formula can be enhanced by the addition of one of the following formulas: *Alpha-curcumone*, an antioxidant formula based on alpha-lipoic acid with curcumin; *Baicalcumin*, a combination of cell-regulating herbs with scute and curcumin; *Genistemma*, a combination for cancer prevention containing soy isoflavones, tea polyphenols, and other flavones; or *Quercenol*, comprising three types of antioxidants—all formulas from the White Tiger brand.

Your pet probably can't get enough phytochemicals from food alone if you are aiming for high quantities. Consuming a wide array of richly colored vegetables and fruits will give your pet a foundation, but he may need to take some of these phytochemicals in supplement form. When considering supplements, look at the link between the type of cancer and the phytochemicals you can use to help keep your pet in remission:

- *Lymphoma:* Isoflavones, vitamin D, and selenium
- *Brain:* Vitamin E complex of both tocopherols and tocotrienols
- *Lung:* Glucosinolates, flavonoids, and vitamins A and D
- *Melanoma:* Flavonoids, vitamins A and D, and curcuminoids
- *Colon:* Glucosinolates, flavonoids, vitamin D, vitamin E complex, and curcuminoids
- *Breast:* Glucosinolates, flavonoids, vitamins D and E, curcuminoids, and lignans

Food sources for the less familiar nutrients are the following:

- *Glucosinolates:* Cruciferous vegetables, such as broccoli, cauliflower, and cabbage
- *Isoflavones:* Soy

- *Curcuminoids:* Curcumin, or turmeric
- *Lignans:* Flaxseed, barley, and quinoa

One last point: it may turn out that the water you and your pet drink could be suspect. Almost all water sources are loaded with pesticides, insecticides, fertilizers, and petrochemicals. Always use filtered water for cooking and drinking.

If you have no access to a filtration system, simply add vitamin C to your water at a ratio of one teaspoon of vitamin C powder per liter of water. This helps ensure that the water maintains an appropriate level of acidity, making it easier for you and your pet to assimilate it.

If you want to go a step further, consider Willard Water as an alternative to your tap. Named after its inventor, Dr. John Willard, this water has a negative charge on its surface that allows it to remove toxins with a positive charge. Willard calls his water catalyst-altered water. This special liquid speeds up chemical reactions without changing their natural results; it is an efficient vehicle for bringing nutrients to cells and carrying away their wastes. Not only is Willard Water appropriate for cooking and drinking, but it is useful for cleaning wounds, treating irritated skin and eyes, and bathing your pet. It's available in concentrated form in several varieties (see appendix D).

Benton became my patient because his human companion and I had clinics in the same building. Benton is a boxer with melanoma. After two operations for tumor removal, when the tumor reappeared for the third time, the owner and I discussed what other options there were. I suggested weekly acupuncture treatments for a month and two herb formulas, *Chih-ku* and *Curcuma* coupled with *Scrophularia* tablets. One is a systemic anti-cancer formula, and the other is a formula specific for soft tumors. For two years, Benton has been doing well on his program. I see him occasionally, and his companion orders his herbs online.

16

RECOMMENDATIONS AND CONCLUSIONS

A much-admired CEO and businessman for four decades, Burton Goldberg, like all of us, depended on conventional medicine when his sister and mother were diagnosed with cancer. Since their deaths, he has spent hundreds of hours and spent $2 million of his own money and gathered together the resources of over 400 practitioners in order to edit and publish the book *An Alternative Medicine Guide to Cancer*. "My interest is in results, so let's get right to the point," he says. "Two systems of health care are available in this country today: conventional Western medicine and alternative medicine. . . . Conventional medicine is superb when it comes to surgery, emergencies, and trauma. . . . But there's no question that alternative medicine works better for just about everything else."[1] His message is simple: cancer can be successfully reversed using alternative medicine.

His book on cancer offers solutions to meeting the challenge of cancer, based on the experience and recommendations of 37 cancer physicians who use complementary/alternative cancer care. These practitioners use integrative oncology in addition to traditional Western methods. In this book, I have presented some of the information and strategies used by these healers and myself in my practice.

None of this information is what you would call new; alternative methods of treating cancer have been with us for decades as adjunct and support. But it was in the 1990s that these approaches moved into significantly wider public awareness. While a great deal of information about alternative approaches is continually being published, most doctors seem to pay no attention, never looking beyond what they have been taught. You are free to take that approach—complete faith in conventional cancer care—and that may be enough to provide good results for your pet. Or you can expand your pet's care to include alternative and complementary approaches that may help restore your pet's health and keep him healthy longer.

Seriously consider the options in this book before making decisions that will have a profound impact on your pet's life. Armed with these data, you can now take control of your pet's care and possibly alter how long your pet will live and the quality of that time. The ideas I've included are some of the best and most successful alternative and complementary health care approaches available right now. And you don't have time to wait. The rate of escalation of cancer cases in pets—in dogs, it's now one out of every two, in cats, one out of three—demands this urgency.

The very first strategy is to consult with your pet's vet and to employ nontoxic treatments first, if at all possible. The idea is to support the patient's own immune capacity to reverse his cancer before the system is practically annihilated by toxic treatments. If you can hold off on conventional treatments, you can improve his chances. Just two or (preferably) three weeks of herbal medicines and/or acupuncture, improved nutritional intake, supplementation, and the like will definitely strengthen his entire body and set the stage for a turnaround. "My belief is that if you intend to cure cancer, you must do more than just destroy the tumor," wrote Dr. Robert Atkins. "The genesis of a tumor is just part of a larger process."[2] What he and, in fact, all such practitioners argue is that the body needs to be rebalanced. If the immune response isn't enhanced, it's rarely possible to achieve a permanent cancer remission.

I like to begin with a wholesome diet. Numerous studies have found that humans who eat plenty of fruits and vegetables have a lower risk of cancer of the stomach, pancreas, colon, rectum, pharynx, esophagus, oral cavity, larynx, lung, bladder, endometrium, cervix, and ovaries.[3] Reviewing studies of dietary influences on these cancers, 80 percent showed a statistically significant protective effect from fruit and vegetable consumption. Why would our pets be any different? Your cat, dog, or bird will definitely benefit when you change his diet to one that includes significant fruits and vegetables. A program of good nutrition, herbs, and supplements will make any further treatment more effective. These are the major steps to take:

- Avoid processed foods—especially the commercial brands of pet food.
- Feed your pet organically raised protein sources—chicken or turkey— with organically grown vegetables and fruit.
- Avoid red meat and chemically preserved foods.
- Plan on a fish meal once or twice a week, such as wild-caught salmon and other oily fish from northern Atlantic sources.
- Supplement a meal with whole grains, such as millet, oats, and other sources of fiber.
- If your cat or dog has never been exposed to fruits, vegetables, fish, or fiber, start with a very low amount and increase it gradually. Your pet may like carrots but not broccoli. Begin there; get him accustomed to those foods he likes, then move forward.
- Another way to put fruits and vegetables into his life is to leave vegetable or fruit drinks out for him in place of his water once or twice a week. Make him a special smoothie or elixir using herbs. Start with very low doses of herbs and gradually move up to a full dose.
- Be sure to include some of the antioxidants suggested. Do not limit your choice to one; they work synergistically, and each has its own specialty.
- Give supplements with meals to promote increased absorption. If you are giving high doses of supplements, divide them into smaller doses and offer them throughout the day.
- Give fat-soluble vitamins, such as vitamin A, the carotenes, vitamin E, vitamin D, and essential fatty acids, such as omega-3, with a meal that contains some fat.
- Give amino acid supplements on an empty stomach. Be sure to use an amino acid blend as opposed to one isolated amino acid. Give a dose of glutathione daily.
- This holds true for the B vitamins as well; be sure to supplement with a complete B complex.
- Give digestive enzymes with meals to aid digestion.
- Add pancreatic enzymes for their use in eliminating toxins; give these between meals.
- Give mineral supplements like zinc and selenium with a low-fiber meal, as fiber can decrease absorption.
- Switch your pet's water to a more purified source.

The herbal foundation of effective cancer therapy has its origins in traditional sources; only recently has this medicine become the subject of intensive, modern research. But herb and plant derivatives are usually slower in onset and less dramatic in impact than those of drugs. As a result, doctors and patients accustomed to the rapid, intense effect of synthetic medicine may become impatient with botanicals.

In most alternative medical centers, botanical agents are used extensively and have been found to work against cancer through several key means: they stimulate DNA repair, produce antioxidant effects, promote production of protective enzymes via indoles (a chemical compound that is an active ingredient), and inhibit cancer-activating enzymes via flavonols and tannins (natural antioxidants). In addition, because cancer patients can die not from the cancer itself but rather from the side effects of conventional treatment, these centers suggest or offer such treatment in smaller doses and at slower infusion rates. The use of chemotherapy is cautious and individualized, generally based on fractionated, or smaller-infusion, dosages administered over an extended period. Such a program not only protects the body but actually enhances the intended effects of conventional treatment. If your pet is to have chemotherapy or radiation therapy, consider asking the oncologist if smaller infusions can be used. Your pet will proceed through the course of treatment more easily.

Within the world of botanicals is the subset of traditional Chinese medicine (TCM) herbal formulas. The herbs used have the backing of modern research, and, because they have an objective track record, they are the ones I almost always recommend. Some of the research results have shown that TCM herbal medicine can effectively complement conventional medicine when the two systems are used in concert against cancer. The *Journal of the American Medical Association* reported that life expectancy doubled for patients with rapidly advancing cancer when specific TCM formulas were added to their treatment plans. The herb-treated cancer patients had twice the survival advantage after one year and four times better survival after two years compared to the chemotherapy-only patients. I have found this same outcome in pets, although there is almost no research to authenticate the results.

In a Japanese study of 260 patients with cirrhosis (a risk factor for liver cancer), half the group was assigned to the combined herbal/conventional treatment, while the other half received only conventional treatment. After five years, 78 percent of the patients in the combined therapy group were still alive compared to 68 percent of patients in the group receiving conventional pharmaceuticals alone. In other studies, survival rates improved in patients with lung, breast, throat, and nasopharyngeal cancer who used Chinese herbs in combination with chemotherapy or radiation versus those who relied on conventional treatment alone.[4]

THE IMPACT OF TOXINS

Ridding the body of its accumulation of toxins is another vital, host-supporting measure. The scale of pesticide residue is staggering: 1.2 billion pounds were dumped on croplands, forests, lawns, and fields according to statistics from 1995—100 million more pounds than in 1993. The National Academy of Sciences estimates that the risk from a lifetime exposure to 28 pesticides in commonly eaten foods could eventually cause 1.46 million additional cases of cancer over the average lifetime. A great number of highly toxic chemicals, materials, and heavy metals are released by industrial processes and find their way into human and pet tissue. They accumulate within the fat cells, central nervous system, bones, brain, glands, hair, and fur. These environmental influences make up one cause of cancers through repeated insults to the body.

Ideally, your cat or dog should go through detoxification on an off-and-on basis throughout his life. If not, and if he has already had conventional treatment, he is probably overloaded with toxins. It would be dangerous to attempt a strong detoxification program at this point. A gentle and gradual workup, particularly of the liver, would be the way to go. An overly toxic liver can be relieved through simple dietary changes, such as emphasizing raw leafy greens and brightly colored vegetables. The use of supplements, such as milk thistle, or a combination of thistle and other botanicals would help the organ. A toxic kidney is another condition seen in cancer patients, particularly in those who have received extensive conventional treatment. Here again, botanicals are the way to go. Reducing the amounts of water-soluble vitamins and amino acids until the kidneys are normal is also indicated, as these nutrients put a strain on the kidneys. A toxic colon may have several causes, including a heavy, meat-eating diet. Abstaining from offering meat to your pet can make an immediate difference. Then, of course, any parasites, pathogens, and so on need to be addressed through herbs and probiotic replacement.

Some additional, general guidelines should be mentioned. Stay away from using aluminum cookware; probably the safest cookware is glass.

Resins in plastic are cancer-causing substances, and the safety of plastics used in storing and cooking various foods, particularly when cooking by microwave, is controversial. Many cleaners—dishwashing liquids, bleaches, scouring powders, and detergents—contain petrochemicals. For your sake and your pet's health, you should take a closer look at what environment he lives in, what you clean with, and what both of you drink. It's almost a sure bet that you will want to make changes once you do so.

An excess of toxins in the environment tends to increase the production of acid within the cells, forcing the body to compensate by producing a strong alkaline chemical reaction in the blood that, in turn, tends to favor the growth of cancer cells. Monitoring for optimal pH by using components of blood, urine, and saliva gives insight into the way the body functions. Making appropriate changes in diet and medical treatment can reestablish health.

A BETTER TOMORROW

A high degree of success in preventing recurrences or metastases of cancer is possible when the inner environment of the body is changed, cells are detoxified, and the immune system is strengthened. Making lifestyle changes beforehand gives the body a head start and prepares it for the stress caused by surgery, chemotherapy, or radiation. I am amazed at the passive attitude on the part of the oncologist and the pet owner toward a cancer patient's future. "The key is to take an active stance against the possibility of recurrences and metastasis, not to succumb to the old wait-and-see policy, which allows these processes to take place and push the cancer out of control," warns Dr. Wolfgang Kostler, president of the Austrian Society of Oncology.[5]

It is a mistake to allow yourself to be lulled into a false sense of security and stop giving supplements, herbs, acupuncture, and the rest to your pet after successfully eliminating much of the cancer. The consequence of returning your pet to his old dietary and other habits is often disastrous. Treating cancer is a lifelong endeavor.

I hope that in the next decade, I see more innovative and effective approaches to the treatment of cancer in animals. So much more can be done. In human cancer treatment, the most promising methods coming out of Europe and the Far East are concentrated in the areas of nutritional substances and homeopathics administered intravenously, individualized vaccines, stem cell therapy, microtumor testing, chemosensitivity tests, genetic tests, and injections of a multitude of supportive and immunity-enhancing agents. I hope that these and other methods of cancer eradication are explored and refined in the United States as well and that our pets can benefit from them too.

Meanwhile, we can work with what is available to us now. We can begin to understand the basics of cancer, and yet, even if its etiology remains largely unknown, we can certainly cut down the incidences of cancer in our pets that result from stresses, chemicals, viral overloads, environmental conditions, nutritional deficiencies, chronic, toxic emotions, chronic diseases, and so on. At the same time, because cancer requires inflammation to grow and spread, we can feed our pets anti-inflammatory foods, antioxidant supplements, powerful enzymes to mop up toxins, and glandular substances to enhance the work of organs such as the liver, kidneys, spleen, and thymus. We can keep our pets' bodies more alkaline than acidic. We can utilize acupuncture and herbal medicines to turn around a weakened immune system. We can take advantage of the many benefits of homeopathy.

You can do this. You can step into the future, and you can help your beloved pet step right there alongside you.

APPENDIX A

Appendix to Chapter 2

CANCER FACILITATORS

Many events take place before cancer actually materializes in form and shape. These events have been researched. Listed below are 33 factors that contribute to cancer, according to a consensus of opinion among researchers and practitioners.[1] Many are interdependent and can form all kinds of combinations. Genetic instability or predisposition combined with environmental causes are together considered to be "precancer event clusters."

Sunlight
Hormone therapies
Parasites
Ionizing radiation (X-rays)
Immunosuppressive drugs
Free radicals
Nuclear radiation
Irradiated foods
Geopathic stress
Pesticides
Herbicides
Residue food additives

Cellular oxygen deficiency
Mercury toxicity
Cellular terrain oncogenes
Sick-building syndrome
Nerve interference fields
Genetic predisposition
Industrial toxins
Polluted water
Toxic emotions
Chronic stress
Tobacco and smoking (exposure to secondhand smoke in homes)
Fluoridated water
Chlorinated water
Miasms
Depressed thyroid action
Diet and nutritional deficiencies
Chronic electromagnetic field exposure
Intestinal toxicity and digestive impairment
Blocked detoxification pathways

Some of these terms may need explanation:

Chronic electromagnetic field exposure consists of long-term exposure
   to electrical currents.
Irradiated foods are those made from substances such as benzene and
   formaldehyde.
Nerve interference fields result from events such as mad cow disease
   (bovine spongiform encephalopathy).
Parasites in this case are primarily viruses.
Cellular terrain oncogenes are those genes that transform from normal
   to abnormal.
Geopathic stress areas are those over the earth's fault lines.

All of the above are considered facilitators of the initiation of cancer.
Excess facilitators can lead to or couple with a weakened immune system,
decrease the removal of free radicals or increase the number of free radicals that the body must deal with, and promote abnormal cell growth. And
bingo—you've got a tumor.

CELL DEATH AND NATURAL AGENTS

Cell death happens through necrosis—exposure to an adverse environment—and through apoptosis—death programmed into the cell at birth and triggered by old age or under conditions where cell death benefits the host. Apoptosis is an orderly method of removing old, damaged, or otherwise unwanted cells (e.g., cell turnover during wound healing). Both processes play a role in limiting tumor growth. Necrosis can occur in cells distanced from a blood supply or as a result of immune activity or even chemotherapy. One possible cause of cancer is the failure of apoptosis to remove cells whose DNA has been damaged. This could allow the cell to survive long enough to progress from initiation to the promotion and proliferation stage. Some cells can even self-inhibit apoptosis. Inducing cell death does play a significant role in limiting net tumor growth.

Natural agents that stimulate apoptosis are the following:

- *Butyric acid:* Formed in the colon by the action of intestinal bacteria on fiber (which may explain the protective effect of dietary fiber against colon cancer)
- *Genistein:* An isoflavone of soy found in legumes
- *Quercetin:* A flavonoid
- *Retinoic acid:* From vitamin A
- *Vitamin D3*
- *Herbs:* Flavonoids and saponins, such as *Scutellaria baicalensis* and *Bupleurum*

ANGIOGENESIS AND NATURAL AGENTS THAT PREVENT IT

Tumors contain an abnormally dense blood vessel network; it's known that tumors induce their own blood supply. The growth of solid tumors is dependent on angiogenesis. Initially, tumor growth is linear before angiogenesis, but it becomes exponential thereafter. Angiogenesis provides tumor cells not only with a blood supply but also with oxygen and nutrients. It also allows tumors a ready access to circulating blood and thus metastasis.

Angiogenesis is a complex process in which existing mature vessels generate sprouts that develop into completely new vessels. The basement membrane surrounding a mature capillary dissolves, and a bud grows out of the capillary. The basement membrane is a layer of specialized connective tissue that the capillary cells are held to. A hollow sprout grows from the bud and migrates, joining its end with another sprout to form a new capillary vessel. There are many angiogenic factors active in tumor growth; interestingly, they are also present in wound healing. That tumor angiogenesis is stimulated by the same mechanisms that are active in normal wound healing suggests that natural agents that affect wound healing may inhibit angiogenesis. Some factors are important to angiogenesis: blood coagulation, inflammation, and tissue repair.

Natural agents that inhibit angiogenesis through a variety of actions are the following:

- Genistein
- *Magnolia liliflora* herb
- Thiol compounds, such as L-glutathione
- Vitamin A
- Vitamin D3 metabolites (these may potentiate the effects of vitamin A and have effects of their own on angiogenesis inhibition)

DIFFERENTIATION AND NATURAL AGENTS THAT INDUCE DIFFERENTIATION

Once a cell becomes neoplastic, its continued replication may result in the formation of a solid tumor. The size of a solid tumor increases because the neoplastic cells within the tumor live long enough for the cell proliferation rate to overcome the cell death rate. Cancers are thought to arise from the proliferation of a single precursor cell: the stem cell. As the initial transformed cell divides and its clones proliferate, individual cells mutate, producing variants of the original transformed cell. This feature allows tumors to adapt more easily to adverse conditions, and some eventually become resistant to chemotherapy drugs.

The progression of some malignancies may be due to a block in differentiation. Agents that induce differentiation can be useful in treating malignancies. When cells are exposed to differentiating agents, they can develop into normal cells and lose their ability to proliferate.

Natural agents that induce differentiation are the following:

- *Berberine:* An alkaloid found in herbs such as *Coptis chinensis*
- *Enzymes:* Bromelain and pancreatic enzymes
- *Butyric acid:* A compound found in the colon resulting from the action of intestinal bacteria (probiotics) on fiber
- *Isoflavones:* Daidzein, found in legumes and soy
- *Docosahexaenoic acid (DHA):* A component of fish oil
- *Ganoderma polysaccharide:* When immune cells are incubated with *ganoderma*, they produce a medium that induces differentiation in cells
- *Retinoic acid:* A form of vitamin A
- *Vitamin D*

APPENDIX B

Appendix to Chapter 4

FEEDING DOGS

A typical dog's diet should consist of about 60 percent protein, about 20 percent vegetables and fruit, and 20 percent grains. For an older dog, adjustments should be made: 35 percent protein, 35 percent vegetables and fruit, and 30 percent grains.

Proteins are essential for growth and development of all body tissues. They are used for the production of enzymes, hormones, neurotransmitters, antibodies, and organ tissues, such as hair or fur, skin, nails, and muscles. Protein deficiency can lead to abnormalities in or lack of development. The type and quality of the protein is directly related to how digestible it is and how well it is utilized. Organically grown meat and wild-caught fish and eggs from organically raised hens are the best sources.

Carbohydrates—vegetables, fruit, and grains—are the chief sources of energy; they convert to glucose, the principal food of the brain, nervous system, and muscles. All animals need them to regulate protein and fat metabolism.

Fats or lipids are the most concentrated sources of energy. They supply more than twice the number of calories per gram as carbohydrates or proteins. Lipids are the main component of cell membranes and are regulators of specific metabolic processes, such as the making of neurotransmitters. Fats also aid in the absorption of fat-soluble vitamins and help make calcium more available.

A dog of 10 pounds needs 400 to 500 calories a day, a 20-pound dog needs 700 to 800, a 40-pound dog needs 1,100 to 1,400, and a 70-pound dog requires 1,750 to 2,000. But remember: one size does not fit all. Keep in mind your dog's age, level of activity, body metabolism, and general health. Particular situations or stages of life also indicate times for adaptation of the diet. Pregnant and nursing moms need more food than usual. Competing and working dogs use more energy and need more calories.

A good way to introduce vegetables to your dog is in the form of broths, soups, or freshly pressed juices in a 50/50 dilution with water. They can be offered in small amounts at first, then gradually increased. With a food-sensitive dog, only one new food ingredient should be introduced at a time, with intervals between foods of several days to determine any possible allergic reaction. The drinks should be pureed and blended.

To extend the storage life of vegetables, put them into a plastic bag before placing them in the "crisper" part of the refrigerator. Pierce the bag in a number of places to allow air to circulate between the bag and the crisper. If left in a bag without air holes, excess surface moisture may form on the produce and hasten its demise.

If you are at a loss on how to start cooking for your dog, here's a simple but hearty beginning recipe; it can be used in place of water two or three times a week or added to good-quality dog food.

HIGH-MINERAL VEGETABLE BROTH

★

This is a recipe often served in health spas, modified from an original recipe by Gayelord Hauser.

1 cup shredded carrots
1 tablespoon chopped parsley

1 quart water
1 cup chopped tomatoes

1 teaspoon honey
1 tablespoon nutritional yeast (optional)

In a large pot, combine carrots, parsley, and water. Cover and cook slowly for 30 minutes. Add tomatoes, honey, and yeast. Let the mix cook for five minutes more. Puree the whole mix in a food processor to make a thick broth drink. Cool and serve. Pour over food, or serve in lieu of water.

Carrots, tomatoes, and parsley give the carotene sources for heart and cardiovascular health and enhance the immune system. The yeast provides a source of B vitamin, and the enzymes in honey activate a number of biochemical reactions associated with digestion. The drink can be served as part of the animal's daily liquid intake and is especially good for an older pet, an ailing pet, a pet with a chronic disease, or a pet with a heart condition. It can also be given to a young pet from a breed with genetic tendencies toward cardiovascular disease (e.g., boxers and papillons).

RECIPES FOR DOGS

If the longevity studies showing that 60 percent of men and 72 percent of women who ate breakfasts every day lived longer are on the mark, the same results should hold true for the dog of the family. A good, hearty, start-the-day meal provides protein for daylong stamina and mental alertness and nutrient-dense carbohydrates for energy, with a small amount of fat and fiber rounding off these much-needed nutrients.

DOGGIE OATMEAL

★

2   cups water

¼   cup sunflower seeds with sesame seeds

½   cup chopped apricots, cranberries, and blueberries,
      either separately or mixed together

¼   cup chopped walnuts with soy nuts

1   cup rolled oats (look for the good, old-fashioned, steel-
      cut variety)

In a one-quart saucepan, bring the water to a boil and add oats gradually, stirring. Reduce heat and cook for about 8 to 10 minutes. Ladle into a bowl and top with seeds, nuts, and fruits. You can serve with a tablespoon of plain, live-cultured yogurt or ¼ cup of soy or rice milk. This recipe makes more than is needed for one breakfast meal. Refrigerate or freeze uneaten oatmeal in single-portion containers. Warm up for a quick breakfast on another day.

In this recipe, the oats are an excellent fiber source for good colon health and also provide the essential fatty acids (EFAs) omega-3 and -6 plus B vitamins. The seeds, nuts, and oatmeal together provide magnesium, zinc, calcium, and potassium, along with vitamin E. Dried and/or fresh fruit provide more fiber. The EFAs, vitamins C and E, and the bioflavonoids from the fruit boost the immune system. Fruit carotenes support artery and vein health. Monounsaturated oils from the nuts and seeds are used by the joints and skin. And the combined mineral content in the recipe is utilized by the bones and teeth, for nerve and muscle stimulation, for slow wound healing (if needed), and for blood clotting. This is an extraordinarily good meal for an older dog or one that has heart or circulation problems, a weakened immune system from a chronic illness, an autoimmune disorder, or high blood pressure or has had a stroke. These ingredients can help slow down aging.

One of the most prevalent and problematic conditions dogs can suffer from is joint changes. Nutrition is important in the treatment of this condition. Tissue repair requires a starting point or a matrix to grow on. Feeding the dog home-cooked food can help slow down the progression of joint degeneration and renew strength and mobility. Stews and soups are an excellent starting place. You can cook large batches ahead and, since they freeze well, serve them all through the week with variations.

All can be made with root vegetables; stock made from bones is a good starting point.

BEEF STOCK

★ ──

Beef or other meat bones
1 tablespoon vinegar

Cook the bones in water over very low heat for an hour with one table-spoon of vinegar, which draws out the minerals. Then discard the bones, and you're ready to start.

For a vegetarian stock, sauté the vegetables right in the pot, then add the water. Cover the pot to bring the liquid to a quick boil, then lower the heat and cook partially uncovered. You will get minimal evaporation and no spillovers. Cook ingredients at a steady simmer. (There will be small bubbles on the surface.) You may take a shortcut by using vegetable bouil-lon cubes as a substitute. Look for no- or low-salt content.

BASIC VEGETABLE STOCK
(THIS CAN BE ADDED TO)

★

1 leek, greens included, cleaned and roughly chopped
2 carrots, slightly chopped

1 zucchini, roughly chopped
2 cups chopped Swiss chard

8 cups water

Place all the ingredients in a large pot or stockpot and bring to a boil uncovered. Lower the heat and simmer for 45 minutes, tasting occasionally. When the flavor develops, remove from heat, strain, and cool.
   You can alter the stock with:

1 celery stalk, roughly cut
1 small sweet potato, peeled and roughly cut

½-inch piece of ginger, sliced into sections
1 tablespoon shoyu

With the vegetable stock made, you can go on to making the actual soup:

VEGETABLE SOUP

★

    4 tablespoons olive oil
1 to 2 pounds (approx.) butternut squash, peeled, seeded, and
           cut into chunks

    2 medium-size sweet potatoes or yams, peeled and cubed
    1 medium parsnip, peeled and cubed

    7 cups stock
1-inch cube peeled ginger (optional)

Warm one tablespoon of oil in a large pot, then add the squash, sweet potatoes, parsnips, stock, and a bay leaf if you wish. Cover and bring to a boil over high heat. Reduce the heat and simmer partially covered for about 20 to 30 minutes. While the soup is simmering, puree ginger in a food processor. Warm the remaining three tablespoons of oil in a skillet and add the ginger. Add this mixture to the soup when the vegetables are cooked. Discard the bay leaf before serving.

SLOPPY JOE

★

1 pound lean ground beef
1 tablespoon chopped garlic

½ cup chopped carrots
1 cup beef-bone broth, made from above recipe

Mix all the ingredients, except for the broth, and place in a frying pan. Cover over medium heat until meat is cooked through. Drain off the fat and add the beef broth, then simmer for 10 minutes, cool, and serve over noodles or other grains.

When cooking stews and soups, start with a large pot with a heavy bottom that prevents scorching. No aluminum. Use cold-bottled or filtered water to make the stock. Avoid hot water because it picks up whatever residue is in the house pipes.

The basic idea behind a good nutrition plan is to stimulate the body's natural cortisone to reduce inflammation and localized swelling in the joints and also to normalize the body's metabolic processes, clean out toxins, and strengthen bones.

DOG TREATS: COOKIES

★

1 cup whole-wheat flour
¼ cup wheat germ
1 teaspoon ginger

½ teaspoon cinnamon
2 tablespoons honey
2 tablespoons molasses
2 tablespoons safflower oil

1 egg yolk

Preheat oven to 350 degrees. In a medium bowl, mix together the flour, wheat germ, and spices. In a small bowl, combine the honey, molasses, oil, and egg yolk. Mix well and add to the flour mixture. Knead dough. Roll out to one-quarter-inch thick and cut with cookie cutter. Bake on ungreased cookie sheet about 15 minutes until lightly browned. Turn off the heat and let cookies dry out in the oven until completely cooled and quite hard.

DOG COOKIES VARIATION I

3 cups whole-wheat flour
½ cup rolled oats

2 teaspoons baking powder
1½ cups milk
1 teaspoon molasses
1¼ cups peanut butter (buy the kind with no sugar and
       preservatives)

Preheat oven to 350 degrees. Combine flour, oats, and baking powder in a large bowl. Using a food processor or blender, mix the milk, peanut butter, and molasses until smooth and add to dry ingredients. Using your hands, knead together. Dough will be stiff. Roll out to one-quarter-inch thickness and cut with cookie cutter. Bake for about 20 minutes or until lightly browned. Turn off the heat and leave the biscuits in the oven until cool.

DOG COOKIES VARIATION 2

★──

2 eggs beaten
1 cup grated cheese (a good cheddar or other hard cheese)

1 cup rice or bulgur, cooked ahead
1 cup vegetables, chopped, grated, or mashed
      (vegetables—peas, carrots, zucchini, yams, and so
      on—can be used singly or together)

1 tablespoon chopped parsley
1 tablespoon nutritional yeast (optional)

Preheat oven to 350 degrees. Blend together and drop by the tablespoon onto a greased cookie sheet. Bake for about 12 minutes or until set and lightly browned. Cool out of oven and store.

Any of these recipes will provide B vitamins, fiber, EFAs, and protein. You can make these treats super-rich by using some spreads.

SESAME AND TOFU SPREAD

★

4 tablespoons soft tofu
2 tablespoons sesame butter or tahini

1 tablespoon honey
1 teaspoon grated orange peel

pinch of cinnamon

Place all the ingredients in a food processor and process. Dab one tablespoon onto a doggie biscuit and serve.

This spread adds crunch and is high in potassium.

OAT BRAN AND TOFU SPREAD

★

¼ cup oat bran
¼ cup soft tofu
1 teaspoon lemon juice

½ banana, cut up
½ teaspoon vanilla
½ teaspoon cinnamon

1 teaspoon grated orange rind

Combine all in a blender or food processor and process until the ingredients are well mixed. Spread one tablespoon onto the biscuit and serve.

FRUIT AND SEED SPREAD

★

1 medium-size eating apple, cut into thin slices
1 tablespoon lemon juice

3 tablespoons soft tofu
1 teaspoon honey

½ cup each sunflower seeds and toasted sesame seeds
½ teaspoon cinnamon

1 tablespoon grated orange rind

Put all the ingredients in a blender or food processor. Process until well blended and smooth. Spread one tablespoon onto the biscuit and serve.

DOG TREATS: LIVER SNACKS

★

Purchase liver from a source that sells organic meats; your dog will be getting the benefits of liver without the liabilities of unwanted hormones, drugs, or other toxins.

Cook the liver in water on top of the stove until done—about five to eight minutes. Drain, cook, and cut into small, bite-size pieces. Put these on a lined baking sheet and place in an oven at 200-degree heat for around two hours or until dried out. The treats can be handed out a few each day or for training or rewarding purposes. Keep covered in the refrigerator.

RECIPES FOR CATS

ROOT VEGETABLES WITH QUINOA

★

This can be a side dish to a good-quality cat food. Fall crops provide the vegetables.

1 teaspoon olive oil
4 medium turnips, peeled and quartered
2 medium-large sweet potatoes, peeled and quartered

¼ cup combination pitted prunes, dried cranberries, and blueberries

1½ cups rutabaga, peeled and diced
1 cup quinoa
1½ cups vegetable stock or chicken stock

1¾ to 2 cups water

Heat the oil in a large frying pan over medium heat. Sauté turnip, sweet potato, and rutabaga for about five minutes, stirring occasionally. Stir in fruit and stock. Bring the mixture to a boil, then reduce the heat. Simmer covered until the vegetables are tender, which is about 30 minutes. Stir intermittently. While the vegetables are cooking, start the quinoa. Put one cup rinsed and drained quinoa in a rice steamer with one and three-quarter cups of water. Cook according to directions for rice. If no steamer is handy, put the quinoa in a pan with two cups of boiling water, cover, and cook over low heat for 15 minutes or until the water is absorbed and quinoa is tender. Fluff up the quinoa and serve with the vegetables.

SWEET POTATO BAKE

★

This can be another side dish, or it can be the main meal—especially for a pet with irritable bowel syndrome.

1 pound soft tofu

2 tablespoons vegetable oil

¼ teaspoon nutmeg

4 medium sweet potatoes, baked

1 teaspoon cinnamon

⅛ teaspoon ginger

Mix all the ingredients in a blender until smooth. Pour into a casserole dish and bake for 20 minutes in a preheated oven at 350 degrees. Cool before serving.

> This is a very digestible dish; the cinnamon provides support for the kidneys and heat to the body, especially for an anemic animal, and ginger is a great energizer for the digestive tract.

SALAD FOR CATS

★

1 tablespoon corn oil
1 tablespoon finely chopped celery

⅓ cup cooked and chopped chicken
2 tablespoons ricotta cheese

2 tablespoons plain, live-cultured yogurt
1 teaspoon brewer's yeast

¼ cup chopped sprouts

Heat the oil in a skillet. Add the celery and cook until soft. Let cool. In a mixing bowl, combine the rest of the ingredients, except the sprouts, and mix well. Stir in the cooled vegetable. Top with the sprouts. Give a small amount if a side dish or a larger amount for the main meal. Refrigerate the rest.

RECIPES FOR DOGS AND CATS

RAINBOW SALAD

★

1 pound firm tofu, cut into ½-inch or slightly smaller slabs
½ pound spinach or egg fettuccine noodles, cooked

1 teaspoon toasted sesame oil
2 cups grated carrots

1 cup grated zucchini or other summer squash
½ cup bean sprouts, rinsed and drained

4 cups finely shredded cabbage

This is a dish of shredded vegetables with bean curd, which can be served as a complete meal or part of a meal. This recipe is also a good, low-protein meal for an animal with kidney issues.

SALMON BURGERS

★

2 cups or about 1 pound uncooked salmon
1 cup cooked wild rice

⅓ cup whole-wheat bread crumbs
1 teaspoon canola oil

The salmon has to be ground. First remove the skin and any bones from the fillets or steaks, then grind in a meat grinder or a food processor fitted with a steel blade.

Mix together the ground salmon, wild rice, and bread crumbs. Shape the mixture into patties. Heat the oil in a frying pan. Cook the burgers until highly browned. Turn them over with a spatula and continue cooking until cooked through. The burgers can be served with plain, live-cultured yogurt and a vegetable side dish.

Salmon ranks near the top in its omega-3 fatty acid content. It provides excellent protein, while the rice is a great source of B vitamins.

RECIPES FOR BIRDS

Cook about two cups of pasta; whole wheat is best. White flour may have added iron, which could lead to iron storage disease. When cool, add about one-quarter cup each of minced broccoli, carrots, green beans, and shredded red pepper. Use a small amount of plain, live-cultured yogurt mixed with crushed walnuts as a dressing. Give a small amount every day.

Birds enjoy many types of noodles, buckwheat and rice noodles in particular. Birds also relish a variety of grains, such as barley, spelt, kashi, couscous, and quinoa, as well as cooked legumes, such as pinto, aduki, and garbanzo beans.

BIRD COOKIES

★ ———

½ cup oatmeal
1 egg with shell

½ cup brown rice flour
4 tablespoons hulled millet

1 teaspoon baking powder (sodium free)
¼ cup shredded or chopped carrots or dried apricots

1 teaspoon vanilla extract
½ cup pureed vegetables, such as a mix of organic yams,
       broccoli, and cabbage

¼ cup 7-grain

Mix dry ingredients together. In another bowl, mix egg and pureed vegetables; stir in dry ingredients just until combined. You may need some water. Lightly butter a cookie sheet and drop by a teaspoon about one inch apart. Bake at 350 degrees for about 9 to 10 minutes. Cool. Keep refrigerated or frozen.

GENERAL TIPS ON COOKING FOR PETS

Meats are either moist-heat cooked or dry-heat cooked. Moist-heat cooking includes boiling, simmering, poaching, stewing, braising, and pressure cooking. Dry-heat cooking includes roasting, baking, broiling, grilling, microwave cooking, pan frying, and deep frying. Young chicken does best in dry-heat cooking, older chicken in the moist-heat method.

It is advisable to cook vegetables in as little water as possible because water will leach out water-soluble vitamins, such as the C and B families. The less water used, the fewer nutrients lost. Steaming food in a scant amount of water and using the leftover cooking liquid as drinking liquid or poured over food are good ways to retain the nutrients.

Cabbage and turnip should not be overcooked. Buy these vegetables when they are young and fresh, and they will not require a long cooking time. If you must buy vegetables from a supermarket, it's probably better to buy them frozen. These vegetables have been frozen within hours of being harvested. The produce is chosen at its best and freshest, and the freezing process is very quick, allowing retention of most of the nutrients.

The following are sources of fiber suitable for pet recipes:

Whole wheat
Peas
Almonds
Parsnips
Carrots
Cabbage
Barley
Green beans
Dried beans
Potatoes
Brussels sprouts
Bran flakes
Citrus fruits
Broccoli
Oat bran
Lentils
Oatmeal
Apples
Spinach
Dried fruit, such as figs and apricots

FOR THE SICK PET: CONGEES

One of the most fortifying and easily digested foods is a congee. Congee is an Anglo-Indian word that means rice gruel or porridge. It is essentially a thick rice soup, with unlimited adaptions and variations. Depending on what is cooked with the congee, it can have many medicinal applications. If your pet is ill from treatment, recovering from treatment, or in poor health before undergoing treatment, a congee is a great tool for rebuilding strength.

A congee can be made from any whole grain: rice, millet, barley, or wheat. The basic idea is to cook the ingredients over hours; the longer the gruel cooks, the more therapeutic it becomes.

BASIC CONGEE

★

1 cup short grain rice
8 cups water

Put the rice in a pot and rinse it under running water to remove any residue. Drain in a colander. Put the rice and water in a heavy saucepan; bring the water to a boil over high heat, uncovered. Reduce the heat to low, partially cover, and simmer for an hour. Stir occasionally.

Additions for extra nutritional effect include the following:

- Carrots, cut, diced, or shredded and lightly cooked, for the vitamin A content
- Ginger, thin sliced, for its curative powers in the case of nausea, diarrhea, and general indigestion
- Pear with a little honey, to cool down the body and bring down a fever, plus help a cough
- Mushroom (made with medicinal mushrooms), for immune boosting.

Once cooked, a congee can be offered with a little milk or honey, or chopped jujubes (Chinese dates).

Herbs can also be added (herbs are discussed in more detail in a later section of this appendix):

- 1 teaspoon dioscorea root
- 1 teaspoon ground codonopsis root
- ½ teaspoon American, Korean, Russian, or Chinese ginseng
- ⅛ teaspoon each of ground cardamom, ground ginger, and ground cloves (for digestion issues)
- 1 dropper *Astragalus* (tincture form), *Ho shou wu* root, and ginseng

All of the above are recommended as tonics to get the patient back to normal. A recovering patient with an appetite can be given a modified congee.

TURKEY CONGEE

★——————————————————————————————————————

1½ pounds turkey bones and parts

2   cups water

3   slices fresh ginger, cut from the root about the thickness
     of a coin and smashed lightly

1   pound turkey meat, trimmed and cut into pieces

1   cup whole-grain barley, rinsed and drained (whole-grain
     barley is more nutritious than the pearl variety)

3   carrots, peeled and diced

3   stalks celery, with ends trimmed and diced

Put the turkey bones, water, and ginger in a large pot and bring to a boil. Reduce heat to low. Simmer for one hour and remove the ginger. Add the turkey and barley to the stock and continue cooking over low heat for about 45 to 60 minutes. Then add the carrots and celery and cook for another 30 minutes. Remove bones.

Traditional Chinese medicine says that the longer the congee cooks, the more therapeutic it becomes. Nuts, such as walnuts and chestnuts, are a good addition and should be added at the beginning of the cooking period with the uncooked grain and water. Vegetables can be either precooked and added at the end or cooked until tender with the rice. For an herbal congee, the herbs should be steeped first in water; then the strained liquid should be added to the cooked congee before serving. Raw herbs can be put into a mesh bag and left in the congee while cooking, then removed and discarded before serving.

MORE RECIPES FOR THE SICK DOG OR CAT

EGG AND LEMON SOUP

★

This is a very light soup; it's very nourishing and easy on the stomach.

> 7 cups chicken broth
> ¾ cup orzo pasta
>
> 3 eggs
> 1 large lemon, juice squeezed
>
> 1 tablespoon cold water

Pour the stock into a large saucepan and add the pasta. Bring to a boil and cook until the pasta is done. Beat the eggs in a bowl until frothy, then add the lemon juice and cold water. Slowly stir a ladleful of the hot chicken stock into the egg mixture, then add one or two more. Return this mixture to the pan and take it off the heat. Do not let soup boil, or the eggs will curdle.

CHICKEN SOUP

⭐

This may get your pet's taste buds going again.

2-inch piece of ginger root, peeled
2½ cups coconut milk

1 cup chicken stock
1¼ pounds boneless chicken breast, skinned and cut into thin strips or diced (for a cat)

Cut the ginger into thin slices. Put them into a saucepan with the coconut milk and chicken stock. Bring to a boil, then reduce heat and simmer over low heat for 30 minutes, stirring occasionally. Add the chicken and simmer for another eight minutes. Remove ginger. Serve when cooled.

TUNA POPSICLES (FOR CATS)

⭐

1 6-ounce can of water-packed tuna
1 teaspoon catnip, crushed fine and organically grown

Drain the liquid from the tuna into a cup with a spout. Fill each compartment of an ice cube tray halfway with water. Lightly sprinkle catnip into each compartment. Fill the rest of tray with tuna water. Place the tray in the freezer and allow cubes to freeze solid.

PUPSICLES (FOR DOGS)

★

    1 quart orange juice
    1 banana, mashed
    ½ cup plain, live-cultured yogurt

Mix all the ingredients in a container with a spout. Pour into empty ice cube trays and freeze.

KITTY MUNCHIES

★

    ½ cup canned mackerel, drained
    1 egg, beaten

    1 cup bread crumbs
    1 teaspoon brewer's yeast

Preheat oven to 350 degrees. Place all ingredients in a medium-size bowl. Mix using a fork. Form the mix into balls about the size of marbles and drop onto a greased cookie sheet. Bake for seven to eight minutes until the balls are golden and crispy. Allow to cool before serving.

WHEN FOOD IS NOT ENOUGH: SMOOTHIES, JUICES, FROTHIES, ELIXIRS, AND MORE

There isn't a single medical system that doesn't have its roots in ancient plant medicines.

Many of our "modern" drugs are derived from or imitate plant substances; indeed, countless medical discoveries have their origins in traditional folk remedies. Yet for many of us, the role of plants in our lives is primarily culinary. Herbs do add eye, smell, and taste appeal to food, but plants are medicines as well.

Modern herbal medicinals are unique in the number of actions they perform: they are pick-me-ups, they detoxify and rebuild all body systems, they calm mental states, and they provide tools for better immunity—altogether, they are a vital part of healing. Taking herbs or giving them to a dog is easy. Smoothies, herbal drinks, and elixirs, combined with fruit juices or broths, are tasty and simple to make. Depending on the effect you want, short- and long-term use of herbs is a safe way to help the body maintain a state of balance and wellness. And adding nutritious drinks to the menu gives your pet more nutrients quickly, so recovery is faster.

The ingredients and equipment required to make simple recipes are fairly easy to come by, and herbal ingredients can be found in reputable health food stores or nutrition centers, by mail, or online. A food processor is a must, but it is only as good as its blades. If you want a machine to perform heavy chores, such as chopping, you'll need a more expensive model with more horsepower. A better processor will have a motor shaft that directly rotates the cutting blade as opposed to a belt-driven model whose belt will keep slipping when you process a heavy load.

Other equipment can include a juicer, a blender, or a handheld, blending wand. A wand allows you to blend one serving at a time right in the cup, glass, or bowl. A press-type and masticating juicer yields a higher-quality juice with more nutrients intact. The drinks should always be freshly packed and consumed within a short time to avoid oxidation and fermentation.

To make, enjoy, and benefit from these beverages, you don't need to turn your kitchen into an apothecary. Begin with simple recipes. The recipes that follow use liquid herbal extracts. This form is superior for use in beverages; it's quick, mixes well, and tastes better than cooked herbs, and the standard dose is usually the dropper that comes with the bottle. Fruits and vegetables in the recipes are chosen for their own medicinal characteristics. You can make substitutions. A few recipes use green super-foods; they are available from reputable suppliers and provide vitamins and enzymes in an easy-to-absorb form, allowing you to add even more nutritional ingredients. Tofu can be used to make a smoothie, as can good-quality, plain, live-cultured yogurt. Both provide protein, if you want an enriched drink. I suggest using alcohol-free herbs, although some products do have alcohol as a base. Alcohol has been used in many of the individual herbs and herbal blends because it is one of the best ways to extract active constituents from plant parts.

Whenever possible, buy and use organically grown herbs and produce. This prevents many chemical residues from ending up in your glass or your dog's bowl. If unsure of the origins of your produce, peel and thoroughly wash items with a vegetable brush. You can also buy washes that will remove most chemical residue. If you are sure that the produce has been organically grown, you can use the skin. Do remove the skin on apricots, grapefruit, kiwi, papaya, oranges, peaches, and pineapple. In some cases, the reason is that the skin may be too bitter, too thick to process, or too toxic. Pits and seeds should be removed. The stems and leaves of most plants can be left intact, except for carrots and rhubarb. Soft fruits that contain very little water need to be pureed in a blender rather than a juicer. The puree is then added to juices. Be sure to use a variety of produce to obtain a range of nutrients.

If you are new to juicing, you might want to try a simple blend until you get comfortable with a juicer. Blend one-quarter each of cucumber, lettuce, and watercress with three-quarters of a tomato. This drink provides lots of minerals. Or you might want to make a simple detoxifier drink to rid the liver and intestines of treatment drugs. You can try a vegetable mix of one part asparagus to three parts carrot or a fruit mix of equal parts of apricot and peach with a tiny amount of grape. Fresh vegetable juices with a small amount of parsley or watercress help to purify the blood. A few drops of fresh lemon juice in water promotes alkalinity and stimulates the enzyme activity of the liver and pancreas. Squeezing the juice from a freshly grated, unpeeled potato is highly effective for helping stomach problems. This juice is rich in enzymes and highly alkaline. Small amounts of cooked red beets and beet greens with carrots produce a juice that benefits the liver and gallbladder. Start with small amounts to test your dog's taste buds.

The following ingredients are listed for their medicinal benefits. Feel free to mix and match:

- Apple: Valuable for digestion and reducing tension
- Apricot: Rich in iron and silicon; useful in anemia
- Asparagus: A powerful kidney cleanser but should be given only in small quantities and always in combination with other ingredients
- Cabbage: Useful for stomach problems, particularly ulcers and lesions, because it metabolizes into vitamin K in the intestines; begin with small amounts and in combinations
- Carrot: Rich in vitamin A and minerals; a good detoxifier and gland stimulant
- Celery: Rich in sodium and chlorine salts; can be used in hot weather to help replace fluids; use in small amounts
- Cherry: Builds blood; rich in iron, magnesium, and silicon; use in small amounts and in combinations since it contains a lot of sugar
- Citrus: Rich in vitamin C and flavonoids
- Cucumber: Rich in minerals, such as sodium, potassium, sulfur, and phosphorus; use sparingly and only in combinations; acts as a diuretic
- Dandelion: Rich in magnesium and iron; a wonderful tonic
- Endive: Add to carrot, parsley, and celery to make an eye brightener
- Grape: Purifies blood, but because it is too sweet in natural sugars for animals, it must be used very sparingly, with other blood-building ingredients; rich in potassium and iron
- Lettuce: Rich in calcium and potassium but should be used only in combinations
- Melon: A good summer drink; a diuretic
- Papaya: Stimulates appetite and aids in digestion; rich in enzymes
- Parsley: Cleanses the body; use in small amounts and in combinations
- Peach: Very alkaline rich and good in diets that call for a pH change from acid to alkaline
- Pear: A diuretic
- Pepper: The green kind; added to carrots, it helps clear rashes thanks to its vitamin C content; use sparingly and in combinations
- Potato: Only used to blend several ingredients together
- Radish: High in potassium; especially good for cleaning and supporting the gallbladder; use in small amounts and in combinations

- Strawberry: Rich in iron, phosphorus, and silicon
- String bean: Stimulates insulin production
- Tomato: Rich in sodium, potassium, calcium, and other minerals; a good source of flavonoids
- Watercress: Very rich in sulfur; use in small quantities and in combinations

Herbal tinctures can be added to juices for specific health issues.

If you are an experienced juicer, you will likely find some new ideas in the following recipes. In any recipe, you can add or subtract herbs and supplements to enhance or change the effects.

ENERGY DRINKS

Everyone wants energy, not just to start the day but also to carry you through—a steady, all-day flow of energy. Pets need this, too.

ENERGY DRINK VARIATION #1

Pour eight ounces of grapefruit juice into a 12-ounce container. Combine with one dropper each of the following herbs: ginseng and *Astragalus* to build energy, *Bupleurum* herb to get the energy moving, and peony herb to get the blood circulating, as well. Add herbal extracts to juice and stir well. You can add three ounces of sparkling mineral water and stir well again.

ENERGY DRINK VARIATION #2— ENERGY AS THE DAY GOES BY

Juice dandelion herbs with a small quantity of parsley and add one dropper of ginger.

ENERGY DRINK VARIATION #3— ENERGY AND LOTS OF MINERALS

Pour eight ounces of orange juice into blender and add one ounce of wheatgrass or green food blend, along with one dropper each of Siberian ginseng, American ginseng, and *codonopsis* herb. Blend until all are dissolved.

ENERGY DRINK VARIATION #4— ENERGY AND BLOOD

Take six ounces of apple juice and add three to five fresh apricots (without pits or skin), several cherries (without stems or pits), and four to five strawberries, all rich in iron. Blend with four to six ice cubes and one dropper each of *Astragalus* and peony. Blend until smooth.

DIGESTIVE DRINKS

Is your pet's digestion off? Here are several drinks for that.

DIGESTION DRINK VARIATION #1

Combine two ounces of papaya juice and six ounces of apple juice with one dropper each of ginger and fennel herbs.

DIGESTION DRINK VARIATION #2

Blend a small amount of cabbage and string beans with one dropper of alfalfa and six ounces of a vegetable-based juice such as "Vedge."

NERVE DRINKS

Are your pet's nerves a bit frayed?

NERVE DRINK VARIATION #1

Put eight ounces of orange juice, one banana, cut into chunks, and one-third of a cup of pineapple chunks, into one-third cup of plain, live-cultured yogurt for a smoothie base. Add one dropper each of schizandra, kava kava, and hops herbs.

NERVE DRINK VARIATION #2

In a small saucepan, simmer eight ounces of apple cider, two droppers of Saint-John's-wort, and two droppers of valerian, with several whole cloves of garlic, one stick of cinnamon, and two to four pieces of fresh or dried orange peel for three to five minutes. Pour into cup and allow spices to settle to the bottom before drinking. Remove all spices before serving to the dog.

NERVE DRINK VARIATION #3

Combine one fresh kiwi, peeled and quartered; one-half cup of fresh pine-apple, chopped; one banana, cut into chunks; four ounces of guava juice; and one-half cup of a sherbet of your choice (pineapple, orange, and so on) with one dropper of ginseng and one dropper of *reishi* mushrooms tincture or a medicinal mushroom combination. (This is a variation of a recipe from "Elixir's of West Hollywood.")

MIND DRINKS

And for your pet's mind.

MIND DRINK VARIATION #1

Mix one cup of fresh blueberries; one cup of melon, cut into chunks; and one-half cup of plain, live-cultured yogurt with one dropper of periwinkle herb, one dropper of gingko biloba, and one dropper of polygonatum herb. Puree in a blender until smooth.

MIND DRINK VARIATION #2

Process small amounts of carrot, parsley, watercress, and celery and blend in six ounces of tomato juice, with one dropper of *Ho shou wu* herb, one dropper of ashwagandha herb, and one dropper of schizandra.

If you are interested in a specific targeted response, choose from several possibilities: among herbs, there is milk thistle for liver support, ligustrum for immune support and cardiovascular health, lycium for the eyes, and honeysuckle for its anti-infective properties. Among foods, try asparagus for the kidneys, cucumber for minerals, pear as a diuretic, pepper to help clear rashes, and radish for the gallbladder.

Many years ago, Adele Davis presented many good ideas on nutrition, and I believe her ideas remain valid today.

PEP-UP

★───

One of her famous drinks is called "Pep-Up," and it attempts to meet the requirements for rebuilding tissue at maximum speed. The drink can be made in the morning in a blender, and small amounts left out for the dog or cat patient.

　　2　egg yolks or whole eggs
　　1　tablespoon lecithin
　　1　tablespoon mixed vegetable oils of sesame, safflower, and olive

　1½　teaspoons calcium lactate
　　½　teaspoon magnesium oxide
　1¼　cups plain, live-cultured yogurt or 1 tablespoon *acidophilus* culture

　1–2　cups whole milk
¼ to ½　cup yeast fortified with calcium
¼ to ½　cup non-instant powdered milk

　　¼　cup soy flour or powder
　　¼　cup wheat germ
　　　vanilla, to taste

To flavor, use vanilla. Blend and pour into a container. Add the remainder of the quart of milk; cover and refrigerate. Stir well before each use. You can add crushed banana or pineapple.

FLAVONOID FRUIT SMOOTHIE

★

A super drink to get flavonoids into your pet's diet is a fruit smoothie; it's easy to make and refreshing to drink.

½ cup sunflower seeds
2 tablespoons nonfat dry milk

1½ cups apple juice, unsweetened
1 medium ripe banana, peeled and cut into chunks

1 medium-size apple, cored and cut into chunks
1 tablespoon plain, live-cultured yogurt

Grind the seeds in a blender. Combine seeds and remaining ingredients in the blender or food processor and whizz until smooth. You can substitute different fruits depending on the season and availability. Use ripe fruits before they spoil.

FLAVONOID FRUIT
SMOOTHIE VARIATION

★

10 strawberries, cut into chunks
1 banana, peeled and cut into chunks

1 peach, pitted and skin removed
½ cup yogurt

1 cup apple juice
1 tablespoon dry milk powder

Combine all ingredients in a blender or food processor. Process until smooth and foamy.

WELL-BEING DRINK

★ ──

½ cup fresh blueberries
1 banana

1 cup apple juice
½ cup silken tofu

2 droppers Saint-John's-wort

This drink will enhance your pet's sense of well-being. In a blender, combine all the ingredients until smooth.

During the late spring, the summer months, and partially into the fall, fresh, local fruits are easy to obtain, and a shake or drink made from these is a yummy substitute for water. Nutrition-wise, the dog will be getting lots of vitamins—especially the carotenes, the C family, bioflavonoids, and antioxidants.

A BERRY GOOD SHAKE

★

½ cup berries, either strawberries, raspberries,
   blueberries, blackberries, or a combination
1 banana, almost ripe

1 peach, ripe
½ cup plain, live-cultured yogurt

1 cup apple, orange, or cranberry juice
2 tablespoons dry milk powder

1 tablespoon nutritional yeast (optional)

To ensure berries are free of toxins from insecticides, pesticides, and fungicides, buy locally from a farmer's market or country stand. Combine all the ingredients in a blender or food processor. Process until smooth and foamy. Serve half one day and half another. Refrigerate leftover portion. You can use this drink as part of the daily fluid intake for a dog.

To really boost your dog's vitality, add one-half to one dropper full of codonopsis root, depending on the size of the dog. One and a half cups of melon pieces, such as cantaloupe, honeydew, or watermelon, is also good. One dropper of the herb *Lycium* fruit extract and one dropper of *schizandra* berry herb tincture will produce a wonderful eye and brain tonic. A shake composed of two ounces of pear nectar and two ounces of kiwi juice, plus one dropper each of *Astragalus*, American ginseng, and *Ganoderma*, kick-starts the day.

DETOXIFYING AND CLEANSING DRINKS

Here are some drinks that are good for detoxifying and cleansing inside the body.

DETOX DRINK #1

★

4 fresh carrots, cleaned but not peeled
1 celery stalk

¼ cup fresh parsley, stemmed
4 ounces chilled tomato juice

Pass the carrots, celery, and parsley through a juicer. Pour into an eight-ounce container. Add the tomato juice and stir to blend.

DETOX DRINK #2

★

7 ounces cooked, peeled baby beets, in natural juice
½-inch piece fresh ginger

2 tablespoons freshly squeezed lemon juice
⅔ cup freshly pressed carrot juice, or the yield from 2
medium-size carrots

⅔ cup freshly pressed apple juice, or the yield from 2
eating apples

Coarsely chop the beet and place in a blender with the juices from the package. Peel and coarsely chop the ginger and add to the blender. Pour in the remaining juices and blend until smooth. Pour into a container and serve at once.

INTESTINAL CLEANSE

Look for a formula that contains aloe, senna, cascara sagrada, barberry root, fennel, and ginger. Any formula should have at least some of these. Also, include ground, organic flaxseed meal.

BLOOD CLEANSE

Look for a formula that contains turmeric, chaparral, yellow dock, thyme, and honeysuckle. Again, be sure these are organically grown.

LIVER CLEANSE

Look for a formula that contains dandelion root, uva ursi, parsley root, and juniper berries. Add wormwood and black walnut in case of parasites and continue with probiotics.

FIBER DRINKS

You definitely want to help your dog ingest a good amount of fiber because of all the good it does. Here are some drinks that will help you do that.

- A smoothie blend of high-pectin fruit: slices of apple, peach, or pear, plus a handful of berries with one-quarter cup of oat bran and one-quarter cup of flaxseed powder. Add a few tablespoons of plain, live-cultured yogurt.
- A mixed-vegetable drink three or four times a week will give your dog his servings of vegetables and will also increase fiber intake. Take one carrot, one tomato, four slices of cucumber, four kale leaves, two sprigs of parsley, three broccoli florets, and a pinch of alfalfa sprouts. Place in a juicer and mix. You can add or subtract different ingredients.
- Mix eight ounces of carrot juice with eight ounces of apple juice and divide over three or more days.
- Twelve ounces of carrot juice with four ounces of spinach juice is another combination.
- Put four fresh carrots, two celery stalks, and one-quarter cup fresh parsley, without stems, in a juicer. Add four ounces of tomato juice. You can also add a thin slice of peeled fresh ginger. This makes a good daily tonic for the dog.
- Whirl 10 ounces of orange juice, one-half cup of raspberries, and one peach, peeled, pitted, and quartered, into one-half cup of plain, live-cultured yogurt until smooth. You can freeze this mix and put it out on a hot day.

APPENDIX C

Appendix to Chapter 11

One of the beneficial strategies you can use to keep your pet healthy is to incorporate herbs in his diet. Keep a few well-chosen herbal extracts or tinctures on hand to use in recipes. Those recommended will be standard tinctures that you can purchase either by phone, mail order, or e-mail from a good supplier, such as those listed in the "Resources" section of this book. It's a good strategy to consult an herbalist, a naturopath, or a practitioner of traditional Chinese medicine (TCM) in difficult, severe, and/or chronic conditions.

To use herbs, you do not need to transform your kitchen into a lab. You may need a few pieces of kitchen equipment to take advantage of their benefits. A juicer not only can save you money but also will extract the maximum amount of nutrients from fruits, vegetables, and herbs for the drinks, blends, juices, and elixirs that you make. You may want a blender to puree ingredients with herbs. A food processor is a great way to mix everything together, ensuring that the dog doesn't pick out the parts he likes and leave behind what he does not. When simmering raw herbs in a soup, wrap raw or dried herbs in a cheesecloth or muslin bag, allowing them to be removed easily before serving.

Herbal ingredients are selected to balance each other. If you live in a big city, you have access to specialty shops and herbal stores, perhaps even a Chinese herb store, for any number of herbs to choose from. When using an herb for the first time, it's wise to give only a few drops just to make sure the patient will tolerate the medicine. Monitor the animal, and if a reaction occurs, discontinue immediately. Then repeat the medicine at a much lowered dose. Be patient. Results will come.

You can help your pet with some of the formulas I suggest and not be concerned about safety. In addition, using liquid herbals makes measuring simple. These products usually come with droppers and directions for the standard adult dose. Adjusting the dose for a pet is simple: for the average dog, it is usually one-half the recommended dose; for small dogs and cats, use one-quarter of the suggested amount.

If there is an underlying digestive problem or weakness, this needs to be addressed first by using one of the digestive aid formulas. Once rectified, you can go on to a new formula. As a rule, animals do well on herbs. When there is improvement, the dose can be lowered and eventually stopped. Administer herbs about an hour after meals rather than on an empty stomach. If any digestion issues arise from the herb use, add citrus peel (lemon or orange), malt, or oryza to the mix.

Introduce a mix of herbs in low doses and, again, monitor the reactions. After two to four days (or several doses) with no unusual reactions, you can up the dose and/or frequency. Many herbs, particularly the tonic herbs for long-range or chronic use, are best given in small doses over an extended period of time. If your pet is sensitive to drugs, he may be sensitive to herbs. Try to use only a few drops at first and build up from there.

RECOMMENDATIONS

Trauma

If your pet has undergone surgery, you can put together an antitrauma compound, one-third each of the following: Arnica root, fresh; Saint-John's-wort flower and bud, fresh; and calendula flower, dried. This group is specific for treating physical trauma. Arnica is traditionally included in most trauma recipes for incidents including shock, coma, and collapse; it promotes tissue repair, reduces inflammation and swelling, and relieves pain. Saint-John's-wort relieves pain and restores injured nerves; this herb reduces contusions, swelling, and pain while promoting tissue repair. Calendula reduces inflammation and swelling, stops bleeding, and also promotes tissue repair. Mix 10 to 20 drops and give at once. Every hour or two, give 5 to 10 drops.

Digestion

Chemotherapy can kill off cancer cells, and antibiotics can destroy bad bacteria, but they can also kill a pet's appetite. Pain and pain medication are also appetite killers. You can help your pet considerably with a few strategies. If your pet has little appetite, try offering very small amounts frequently throughout the day. Offer snacks, such as biscuits with nutritious tasty spreads. Try soft, cool foods, such as a shake or a smoothie. Try soups, stews, or chowders instead of regular solid food. Definitely dose him with alfalfa. And you can make a digestive aid mix of herbs.

One-third each of meadowsweet flowers, fresh; chamomile flowers; and fennel seed are ingredients that soothe an overactive digestive tract; ease gastritis, heartburn, and dyspepsia; and relieve nausea. Meadowsweet acts on conditions aggravated by heat and soothes the inflamed mucous membranes of the digestive tract. Fennel refreshes, comforts, and strengthens the stomach. This formula can be used when traveling with pets. Use as needed in an acute situation. Dose is three to eight drops.

Another formula aimed more for reestablishing an appetite is digestive bitters: equal amounts of fresh dandelion root, fresh peppermint rhizome, centaury herb, gentian root, and ginger rhizome. This formula stimulates the entire digestive system, helping in the absorption of nutrients and the elimination of toxins. It can be used as a tonic through the action of gentian and dandelion. The formula stimulates digestive enzymes as well as bile production. Symptoms of gas, belching, congestion, indigestion, and malabsorption are all covered. This is the kind of formula you can build on by adding herbs to address specific concerns. Fennel can be added for flatulence, cardamom to stimulate additional digestive enzymes and saliva production, rosemary to calm down spasms, or angelica to relieve fullness and stool mucus. Give 2 to 10 drops in a small amount of warm water 15 to 20 minutes before meals. This formula is safe to use over several months to rebuild a poor digestive system.

Nausea and Vomiting

Nausea and vomiting are very common to chemotherapy patients. Many chemotherapy agents are notorious for causing nausea and vomiting. The herb ginger is an effective antiemetic therapy and can be offered as a tea or a supplement. You can buy ginger root, keep it frozen, and, when you need it, simply cut several thin slices and steep in hot water. Allow to cool and serve. Again, offer only small amounts of food throughout the day. In these cases, hot cereal, a congee, or a soft-boiled egg are easily tolerated.

Ice chips, plain or sprinkled with a little salt and fruit juice, will help keep your pet hydrated and his electrolytes balanced. If your pet becomes severely dehydrated, you may have to hydrate him with fluids obtained from your veterinarian. You can purchase a special hydrating saline formula called Ringer's (with its accompanying setup) at your veterinary clinic. Have the process explained and demonstrated so that you can repeat it at home. You can also feed your pet electrolyte-restoring drinks, such as children's formulas. Avoid feeding the animal any strong-smelling, fatty, or spicy foods.

Diarrhea

Your pet can develop diarrhea as a result of chemotherapy, radiation to the abdomen, an infection picked up in a hospital, antibiotics, or other drugs. Diarrhea can lead to dehydration and nutrient malabsorption because the partly digested food is moving too rapidly through the system for the intestines to absorb its nutrients. Avoid serving any foods that could speed up peristalsis, such as fatty foods, spicy foods, acidic foods, and raw fruits and vegetables. High-fiber food, such as brown rice, can be offered in limited quantities. Diarrhea-fighting foods include porridge, congees, barley broth, and tapioca. If your pet has an appetite, give him fish (instead of meat), banana, and potato—all good sources of potassium. Once you get the diarrhea controlled, slowly reintroduce easily digested food, such as vegetable broths, grated apple, steamed carrots, and rice or barley cooked in twice the usual amount of water so that it becomes a thin porridge. Supplements that might help are glutamine, 1 gram twice a day; quercetin, 250 milligrams two to four times a day; and, of course, probiotics.

Constipation

Constipation in animals can be dangerous because fecal impaction (feces collecting in the lower colon) can be fatal. Constipation for cancer patients may be a side effect of pain medication, a low-fiber diet, lack of physical activity, or low fluid intake. Try to have your pet drink more water daily. Sprinkle a tiny bit of salt in his food so he will be thirsty. Increase his fiber intake with a variety of fruits and vegetables (e.g., apples and bananas contain pectin, a water-soluble fiber). Mix seeds such as flaxseed, sesame, and sunflower, along with sprouts, such as alfalfa, into his food or prunes soaked in water. Increase the intake of high-fiber foods gradually. Herbs that are useful are senna, cascara sagrada, and whole aloe leaf. One capsule before bedtime can stimulate the next day's movement.

Sore Mouth

A sore mouth can afflict up to 40 percent of chemotherapy or radiation patients. The condition called mucositis can involve mouth sores, painful or dry mouth, or burning, peeling, or swelling of the tongue. The condition can be treated from several diverse angles: homeopathic mercury, 30c or 200c, three pellets dry, two or three times a day; the amino acid glutamine, 2 grams mixed in a bottle of water and swished or sprayed into the mouth every hour; the herb licorice, or aloe vera gel, swabbed on the gums with vitamin E, three times a day; or mix slippery elm or marshmallow root in the daily water.

Bladder and Urinary Tract Issues

Several other herb formulas can help with issues that arise from conventional treatment. Bladder and urinary tract problems can come up because of drug therapies, including pain medication, antibiotics, or steroids. Mix equal parts of cleavers, fresh; pipsissewa herb; corn silk; uva ursi leaf; and horsetail shoots. Cleavers is a diuretic good for an irritated and inflamed bladder. Combined with corn silk, the two are used for cystitis, nephritis, and urethritis. Horsetail is another diuretic useful for urinary tract infections, especially with bladder inflammation and blood in the urine. Pipsissewa and uva ursi are antiseptics for cases of burning and painful urination. This formula can be enhanced with juniper, a very strong antiseptic; marshmallow, which soothes and cools the urinary tract; couch grass for its antimicrobial value; and goldenrod for an infection—10 to 25 drops in water, three to five times a day, for an acute condition. This formula can be used in conjunction with any antibacterial program for speedier results. Or mix one-quarter parts of black walnut hulls, fresh; elecampane root, dried; sweet annie herb or artemisia leaves and tops; and wormwood leaves and tops. These ingredients are antifungal and antiyeast agents and can be given for four weeks and then stopped.

Respiratory Ailments

For lungs, try equal amounts of elecampane root; hyssop parts; coltsfoot leaf, fresh; and bee pollen. This formula is helpful for relieving any distress from respiratory ailments; it works on soothing and toning the lungs, relieving irritation, and aiding as an expectorant. Elecampane builds up lung energy, and hyssop, coltsfoot, and thyme calm a cough, reduce mucus, and act as antimicrobial agents. Give three to five drops in water, three times a day, as needed. Discontinue after four weeks.

Eye and Ear Problems

An herbal eye wash soothes and cleanses burning eyes and irritation from conjunctivitis. Try one-quarter portions of eyebright flowering herb; mullein flower; rue tops, fresh; and goldenseal root and rhizome, dried. Place 3 to 10 drops in a small container and fill with saline solution (salt and water). Stir until well mixed, then use as a wash, for approximately one to two minutes for each eye. Repeat up to three times a day if needed. Try to keep the eyes open while administering. If the wash seems too strong, lower the number of drops. Or begin eye care with three to five drops and add more drops when tolerated. A small bottle is ideal for making and keeping unused portions of the mix. The liquid can be carefully poured out, and the bottle will not be contaminated.

Herbal ear drops can be made from one-third equal parts of calendula flower, dried; mullein flower, dried; and garlic bulb, fresh, in tincture form. These ingredients inhibit and destroy bacteria, fungus, and yeast in the ear canal. They also work on inflammation, itching, and pain. For acute infections, congestion, and inflammation, place one or two drops into each ear, two or three times a day, and massage the ear. Make sure the dropper doesn't come into contact with the ear or fur or other sources of contamination. Never place cold drops into the ear; hold the bottle between your hands for a few minutes to warm the oil.

Mind and Spirit

Several herbs act as nerve restorers and mind/spirit relaxants. Their main effect is on fatigue, anxiety, restlessness, pain, stress, and the inability to sleep. Mix one-fifth each of skullcap flowering herb, fresh; oat berry, seed or straw, fresh or dried; avena sativa; lavender flower, dried; melissa leaf, dried; and rosemary, dried. Rosemary is beneficial for general debility from a chronic illness. Skullcap promotes rest. Lavender helps during recovery from a prolonged illness, calming the spirit, reducing a fever, and, in general, relieving anxiety. Avena is nourishing in general. This compound serves to restore the entire nervous system and speed up recovery from an illness. Give 10 to 20 drops in water, three times a day, and save the last dose of the day for before bedtime.

All of the above formulas are based on the assumption that you will buy the raw herbs and brew the mix, but you can buy each herb in a tincture form (liquid) and mix the liquids together. You can also buy a comparable formula mix from any of the companies listed in the "Resources" section of this book. Any of these approaches will get you results.

Additional Formulas

- One dropper full of polygonatum helps support the body; when combined with gingko biloba, it supports the mind. For an overworked or overstressed dog, it will clear the mind and restore normalcy.
- One dropper full of damiana for fatigue.
- One dropper full of gota kola for a dog who is off balance. Often used for pain, dehydration, summer prostration, and even hysteria.
- One dropper full of hops for a good night's sleep. This herb calms and mellows the dog; adding a little honey to it counteracts the bitterness.
- One dropper full of Saint-John's-wort for the slightly depressed dog. This herb can be given internally and also applied as a massage oil for its traditional use in alleviating neuritis and neuralgia pain.
- One dropper full of mint for cooling down a pet. Mint freshens the mouth, and, because it is cooling, it can be used in the drinking water through a hot, humid day.
- One dropper full of zizyphus for restlessness at night, a wonderful sedative for any nervous condition.
- One dropper full of valerian for the anxious dog. This herb has an antispasmodic and calming effect.
- One dropper full each of ginger and licorice to aid the digestive tract.

Herbs need to be used on a consistent basis. For example, with an older dog that is very restless at night, zizyphus would need to be used daily for two to four weeks to achieve results.

ANTITUMOR EFFECTS OF SOME CHINESE HERBS

Studies have confirmed that a number of Chinese herbs have anticancer properties:[1]

1. They inhibit invasion.
2. They inhibit angiogenesis.
3. They induce apoptosis.
4. They are cytotoxic.
5. They inhibit metastasis.
6. They induce differentiation.
7. They stimulate the immune system.

Here are some of these herbs:

- *Acanthopanax*: Its polysaccharides inhibited tumor growth by up to 67 percent and prolonged survival by up to 71 percent. Up to 33 percent of the mice studied experienced complete remission.
- *Angelica sinensis*: Its polysaccharides increased the life span of fibrosarcoma-bearing mice by up to 170 percent.
- *Artemisia capillaris*: Showed direct cytotoxic action with no associated immunosuppression.
- *Astragalus membranaceus*: Improved the function of T-lymphocytes in human patients by 260 percent.
- *Cordyceps sinensis*: In treated mice, macrophage activity increased to levels approximately four times greater than in the control group. In other experiments, macrophage activity was restored to normal levels after being suppressed.
- *Curcuma aromatica*: It exhibited marked antitumor activity.
- *Ganoderma lucidum*: Increased life span up to 195 percent. Its antitumor action is believed to occur through T-cell activation.
- *Panax ginseng*: Reduced tumor weight by as much as 75 percent, inhibited metastasis, and decreased the elevated platelet and fibrinogen levels induced by tumor cells.
- *Scutellaria baicalensis*: Produced a normalizing effect on hemostasis; this activity may be responsible for the herb's metastasis-inhibiting effects.

There are many wonderful TCM herbal formulas to which you can turn if your pet is ill. One such group I can recommend comes from the White Tiger brand, another from Seven Forests, and others from Health Concerns. The goal of these formulas is to manage the full range of supplements a patient might be taking—including Western vitamins along with herbs—and to integrate TCM herbs with Western methods of treatment. As a result of the ongoing interchange between Western and Chinese medicine, there has been a great deal of cross-pollination of the two types of styles in China today. Clinical use has been further transformed by research and publications on therapeutic regimens combining the modern and the traditional.

These formulations integrate highly concentrated vitamins and minerals as well as nutrients from plant constituents and active ingredients, such as those from the flavonoid family. These products are nontoxic and can be used without extensive medical training:

From the White Tiger Brand

- *Cartaequin:* A formula for improving circulation and cardiac function, which includes many of the recommended supplements for heart problems: coenzyme Q10, vitamin E, and the hawthorne herb. The formula is very useful for certain breeds, such as boxers and papillons, and those that tend toward cardiovascular problems.
- *Galletaine:* A formula providing digestive enzymes for indigestion, malabsorption, poor appetite, low body weight, and many digestive processes as a result of aging, chronic disease, or long-term poor diet. It further includes betaine HCL and traditional herbs.
- *Gincofolin:* A combination of herbs and nutrients to promote nervous system health, Gincofolin can be used for improving circulation to the brain since it provides brain food, such as choline, lecithin, and inositol.
- *Iron Shougui:* An iron supplement with minerals and organic acids to improve the absorption of the iron. This is a good addition to the life of a pet in renal failure or one that is suffering from liver disease or general poor health. It can be used over a long period of time with no adverse effects.
- *Lycuvin:* Herbal extracts plus flavonoids from bilberry and lutein, this formula works to prevent vision problems associated with aging. Can prevent cataracts and slows down other degenerative conditions.

- *Propol-Gold:* This product is a general, first-aid, antiseptic blend of herbal substances, particularly flavonoids, that inhibits a wide range of infections—bacterial, viral, yeast, and fungal. The ingredients are natural nutrients for treating infections of either a topical or a systemic nature. It can be given in tandem with an antibiotic and enhances the antibiotic's overall effect.

From the Seven Forests Brand

- *Astragalus 10+:* Enhances immune system functions.
- *Bidens 6:* For viruses and acute or chronic problems.
- *Blue Citrus Tablets:* Adjunct therapy for breast and liver cancer.
- *Chih-ko and Curcuma:* Treats solid cancers, typically paired with other formulas, according to cancer type.
- *Clear Heat:* For viral, bacterial, and fungal infections.
- *Zedoaria:* For abdominal masses.
- *Viola 12:* Treats toxic swellings.
- *Ganoderma 18:* Enhances immune functions.
- *Gynostemma Tablets:* Used as an adjunct to other cancer therapies; very useful in boosting energy before the use of conventional medical therapy. Should use for four to six weeks after intensive medical therapies are concluded.
- *Paris 7:* Prevents activation of dormant DNA disease strands.

From the Health Concerns Brand

- *Regeneration:* Contains herbs thought to have an antitumor effect, based on Chinese research.
- *Coriolus PS:* Japanese research shows medicinal mushroom extracts have antitumor effects, stimulating natural killer cells and tumor necrosis factor.
- *Serramend:* Dissolves necrotic tissue and blood clots and supports the breakdown of fibrin.

GENERAL TIPS

Using herbs does require some basic information. If buying them on your own, choose a company known for its serious commitment to herbs. This ensures herbs that are grown in the cleanest areas, free from environmental toxins, and processed with good quality control. Herbs in their natural form contain hundreds of active constituents. Yet most companies manufacturing herbs use standardization, an attempt to produce one major, active ingredient that is considered responsible for the health benefit. This marker serves as a standard measure for potency, but it leaves open this question: What of the other 99 active ingredients? Moreover, herbs like to work together, helping each other achieve their range of benefits.

It's important to use herbal products responsibly. Herbs have both a traditional and a modern application and have an accepted range of benefits through proper use. Tonic herbs (as in the drink recipes provided earlier in Appendix B) are considered more nutritive than therapeutic and are, on the whole, safe to use as an adjunctive course. But do your research. Do be wary of advertising claims. Do follow the directions on the label. If you have a particular objective, seek professional advice.

APPENDIX D

Appendix to Chapter 13

ADJUSTING THE PH OF YOUR PET

If your pet needs more of an alkaline environment, include some of the following foods in his diet:

Alkaline-Forming Foods

Alfalfa (and other sprouts)
Apples
Apricots
Asparagus
Bananas
Beans (lima, and green types)
Beets
Berries (except blueberries and cranberries)
Broccoli
Brussels sprouts
Cabbage
Cantaloupes (and other melons)
Citrus
Dates and figs

Eggplant
Grains (millet, quinoa, and amaranth)
Honey parsnips
Peas
Potatoes (with skins)
Pumpkin
Sea vegetables
Soy
Spinach
Squashes
Tomatoes (vine ripened)
Yams and sweet potatoes

The following foods should be avoided if you want to increase the al-kalinity of your pet's internal environment or added if you wish to do the opposite:

Acid-Forming Foods

Beans (dried: lentils, chickpeas, garbanzo)
Blueberries and cranberries
Cheese
Cottage cheese
Egg whites
Fish
Meat (all)
Prunes and dried fruit

Extra-virgin olive oil and other fresh, cold-pressed vegetable and seed oils are considered to be neutral.

Make a diet of 35 percent vegetables and fruit. As much as possible, give this food to your pet raw, such as apple slices, bananas, pear pieces, carrots, and so on. One such meal would consist of sliced apples, half a ba-nana, cooked pumpkin or squash, and 60 percent cooked chicken and the remainder rice or wheat. Or you could do 50 percent cooked carrots and broccoli, with salmon and rice making up the other 50 percent.

ALLERGIES

Allergies are one example of a health problem that you can treat and even prevent through diet and supplementation. If your dog is plagued with chronic itching, foul-smelling bowel gas and stool, infected ears with a smelly discharge, chronic indigestion, pasty gums, or irritability or is constantly licking between his toes and/or chewing on parts of his body, these symptoms may be manifestations of a high toxic load, concentrated in the intestines.

Conventional medicine treats allergies with drugs, but the response is often short-lived. The steroids or antibiotics that are used will cause skin eruptions, for example, to disappear, but they are just as likely to push the problem deeper into the body. With repeated rounds of eruptions and treatment, the problem becomes much more difficult to cure. What started as an acute allergic response some time in the past lasting for a short time now develops into a condition lasting months, even all year. And the dog is an unhappy creature.

The good news is that there's a much simpler and benign—not to mention more effective—way to calm and cure allergies. Instead of adding drugs, you can begin at the problem's source: reducing the toxins in the dog's food, body, and environment. Begin the treatment with a day of fasting in which you provide your dog with nothing but good water (like spring water or Willard Water). Use glass or a stainless-steel container for a water bowl to further ensure that no chemicals leach from plastics. A fast will allow the bowels to clear, and the water intake will begin flushing out toxins.

On the second day, offer your dog only a few foods that are unlikely to cause food allergies. The diet should have no cereals, no dairy, no processed foods, and no sugars. The food at this point should have more protein than carbohydrates. It should be chemical free, organic, and cooked at home. Chief ingredients can be free-range, organically grown beef or poultry raised on food sources free of antibiotics and hormones. Fish, such as wild salmon or cod, are acceptable. Fruits and vegetables should be peeled and washed, having been bought from organically grown sources. All ingredients should be lightly cooked.

The diet I recommend is the Rotation Diet, introduced by Dr. Herbert J. Rinkel in 1934 for his human patients and adapted here for dog patients. Rinkel suggested starting with a small group of easily tolerated foods. You can offer your dog a different diet each day for four days. After each day, observe any reactions from these specific foods either in his elimination, on his skin, or in his general well-being.

The diet goes something like this:

Day 1
Chicken or turkey; carrots or parsnips; banana

Day 2
Fish, wild, fresh cold-water type; a legume, such as lentils, cooked; pumpkin; zucchini or other squash

Day 3
Eggs; tomato and asparagus; apple; tapioca, cooked and mixed into food

Day 4
Greens, such as cabbage, broccoli, or Brussels sprouts; yam or sweet potato; barley, oats, millet, or soy; whole-wheat or vegetable pasta; plain, live-cultured yogurt

After the first cycle is completed (days 1 through 4), go back and repeat the rotation again for another four days. After two, three, or even four rotations, you can gradually start reintroducing other foods into the diet. For example, if you used carrots on day 2, you may add or substitute parsnips for the carrots. The day 2 menu can have two members of the squash family and a different legume. In the day 4 menu, you can add a leafy green vegetable.

If the gastrointestinal system is rested for a short time, then it is usually able to repair itself. Your dog will tolerate almost any food if it's introduced in this way.

CLEANING THE INSIDE

The problem of toxic overload has grown significantly, as the number of toxic compounds in food, water, and the environment has increased in multiple quantities. The overall health of a body is severely influenced by the volume of these toxins taken in and the body's ability to get rid of them.

Every year in the United States, manufacturers, power plants, motor vehicles, and other polluters spew out some of the most toxic chemicals known. The Union of Concerned Scientists estimates that in the food supply alone, the residue of 24.5 million pounds of antibiotics is fed to farm animals. Humans, who are above these animals in the food chain, ingest the residual medical toxins with each meal. There is no one alive today who does not have polycyclic hydrocarbons in his or her fat tissues. Research suggests that up to 90 percent of all cancers begin when the amount of environmental carcinogens overwhelms the body's detoxification ability.

Waste products and cellular debris formed in the body are another kind of serious pollutant and can cause significant alterations in body functions. These continual buildups in the colon are linked to many illnesses, among them diabetes, colitis, thyroid problems, allergies, asthma, liver disease, pancreatitis, autoimmune diseases, and cancer.

Toxins are dealt with in two ways: they are excreted through the elimination organs (the lungs, intestines, skin, liver, and kidneys), and they are neutralized by the macrophages (members of the white blood cells). Effective elimination lies in all these systems working up to capacity.

The major player in the process is the liver, for it copes with the myriad chemicals that pass through it on a daily basis. A healthy liver goes through two phases in the detoxification process. Phase I employs a group of 50 to 100 enzymes referred to collectively as P450. Each one of these enzymes is selective about which target chemicals it goes after, but there is considerable overlap. How diligent and thorough these enzymes are depends on genetics, the levels of toxicity already present, and the body's nutritional status. A body in which these enzymes are working efficiently is unlikely to succumb to major health problems. In contrast, a body with underactive enzymes will show symptoms of digestive disorders, skin problems, allergies, and organ system disease.

There is a catch to phase I detoxification. Each time the liver reduces a toxin to a water-soluble substance and neutralizes it, the organ eliminates one threat but creates another, called free radical by-products. Decades ago, Dr. Denham Harmon, a medical researcher and practitioner, theorized that free radical reactions could be responsible for the progressive deterioration that typically accompanies the aging process. A free radical is essentially an atom or group of atoms with at least one unpaired electron. The free radical tries to steal an electron from a normal cell (it is highly motivated to do this), and the normal cell is irreversibly damaged.

Under this theory, reducing free radical damage is one very important solution to disease and aging. The important requirement for an effective

P450 phase is the reduction of free radical by-products. The job gets done through the action of the amino acid glutathione. Glutathione is a protein produced in the liver from three other amino acids: cysteine, glutamic acid, and glycine.

Glutathione plays a large role in cellular protection; the rate at which a body ages is directly correlated with glutathione concentrations in cellular fluid. This nutrient has many more benefits: it has anticancer and detoxification effects, reduces toxic side effects from conventional therapies, synthesizes proteins, repairs DNA, protects enzymes, restores other antioxidants, and regulates apoptosis and cellular differentiation on at least 12 carcinogens identified as being susceptible to attack from glutathione. In 1974, researchers demonstrated the ability of glutathione to kill neuroblastomas and cervical carcinomas. In 1983, further research showed that glutathione was capable of destroying leukemia cells. Further research in 1988 and 1993 showed that glutathione inhibited tumor progression and transformation of precancerous cells into malignant cells in several types of cancer: liver, skin, mammary, oral, and pharyngeal. In 1997, studies reported the successful use of this supplement on polymetastasized cancer, extending quantity and quality of life.[1]

Certain foods enhance phase I detoxification: these are members of the *Brassica* family, such as cabbage, broccoli, and Brussels sprouts. Citrus foods, such as oranges and tangerines, are great detoxifiers as well since they break down to the active chemical limonene, which blocks carcinogen activation and tumor growth.

Phase II continues the detoxification; its activity depends on having adequate supplies of the thiols, or sulfur-containing amino acids. When both phases are completed, the neutralized toxins need to be excreted. Bile, stored in the gallbladder and secreted by the liver, helps this process. But the flow of bile can be hampered by the presence of gallstones, gravel, inflammation, and lesions.

During day-to-day detoxification, bulk fiber and lots of water are important to help clean properly. Because it is indigestible material, fiber scrapes along the intestinal walls, pulling out longstanding fecal matter, and pushes all this debris out with the stool. Fiber comes from fruits and vegetables and gummy carbohydrates, such as oatmeal and oat bran.

Membranes of the liver cells have as their main component phosphatidylcholine, or lecithin. Stability, health, and resistance to infection, and other assaults on these membranes are directly dependent on their lecithin content. Supplementation with lecithin restores the proper amount of fluidity to these membranes, enabling them to function more normally again. The numerous viruses that damage liver cells have lipid envelopes, or outer coatings. The lipid envelope viruses include some of the most dangerous viruses known, including hepatitis, the whole family of herpes viruses, HIV in humans, and FIV in cats. If the fluidity of these viral membranes is increased, these viruses become destabilized and inactivated. Lecithin alters the membrane of the virus, making it less infective.

Lecithin has proven to be useful in detoxifying even some of the most severe side effects of neuroleptic drugs. The ability of lecithin to purge the cells of rigidifying cholesterol is a profound antiaging effect. In research, it's been shown that liver cells of old animals could still be fluidized by giving supplemental oral lecithin, returning those cells to a condition closer to what is normally seen only in younger animals.

A dog (or human) with hepatitis, liver or kidney disease, digestive problems, skin issues, allergies, and so on has a compromised body. Such a case needs a liver flush. This is made from carrots, beets, and a small amount of celery juiced together, used daily for a week, and then stopped. Bulking agents, such as mucilaginous herbs, along with a small amount of aloe vera and daily probiotics, should be included in the regimen.

Herbs are a great way to clean organs and body systems. In the case of the liver, members of the thistle family with the active ingredients of silymarin and silybin are singularly effective in treating liver damage. Milk thistle herb and artichoke herb can stop liver damage by acting as free radical scavengers and stimulating liver cell regeneration. A series of studies found that silymarin fosters regrowth of cells when part of the liver is surgically removed. Biopsies have shown that this herb is effective in treating both acute and chronic viral liver disease. These thistles are low in toxicity and are tolerated well. They need to be used for very long periods of time in severe liver damage. Milk thistle and artichoke have to be used with glutathione because large numbers of free radicals will be generated in the cleaning process. These by-products will be dumped into the intestines and will use up all available amounts of glutathione. So supplementing with additional glutathione is a must.

Among all the thistle family herbs, artichoke is the top choice if digestion is poor because the liver is not producing enough bile. The herb helps with dyspepsia, severe constipation, and colic. It will stop vomiting, diminish abdominal pain, improve appetite, and reduce gas. Artichoke also relieves irritable bowel, altered bowel functions, excessive secretion of mucus in the colon, and general low-grade nausea and malaise.

Bitter herbs, such as dandelion root, can boost a sluggish liver and can be incorporated into a diet plan for a month or two. Oregon-grape root herb helps control bile production and slows the transit time of bile through the intestines. Slower transit time ensures good breakdown and absorption of nutrients as well as more thorough elimination through the colon.

A dog can benefit from a detoxification once or twice a year. Here's how it works. First, no food for a short period of time, usually one day. The fast has to be helped with plenty of water, fruit drinks, or vegetable broths. Add glutathione because the depletion of the body's stores of amino acids will lead to free radical havoc. After the initial fast, the next step is a modified food fast for approximately three to five days. A three-day program is enough for a healthy body. A longer program is appropriate for one who has never been on a detox or who has allergies or skin issues. Food intake consists of a whole-grain, cooked organic chicken; a vegetable; and a portion of fruit. A high-quality multivitamin and mineral supplement—without iron but with selenium, zinc, and copper—is a good addition. An even more comprehensive approach is to add extra vitamin C, a multicarotene, an amino acid mixture, and extra herbs. Milk thistle, dandelion, artichoke, parsley root, burdock herb, and horsetail herb are excellent additions, as is S-adenosylmethionine (SAM-e), a sulfur derivative helpful in treating bile stagnation and increasing the flow of bile.

The last part of the process is the recolonizing of the intestines with beneficial flora, the probiotics, which will change the pH balance, making the environment slightly more acidic and discouraging the growth of unfriendly bacteria, yeasts, and viruses. Once cleaned out and repaired, the body will start rebuilding itself.

It has been my experience that turning the liver around takes months, so I caution clients that we could end up with any of three different scenarios when the next set of laboratory readings is done. The lab readings could go higher—either an indication of steady regression into the disease or simply a sign that the alternative treatments haven't had time to work. The readings could go lower. Or they could stay pretty much the same. Either of these last two possibilities would show that the condition was responding to treatment.

CLEANING THE OUTSIDE

Brushing your cat or dog daily is actually another way to keep him healthy. Pay particular attention to areas where the lymph system is prevalent: all four legs at their inside attachment to the trunk, along the collarbone, and in the sternum and rib cage connections. This helps lymph fluid move toxins out of the body more efficiently. Use a moderately soft, natural vegetable fiber bristle brush. Synthetic fibers tend to build up static and magnetic energy in addition to being too sharp. Wash the brush every couple of weeks with soap and water and dry before using. This will get rid of any impurities picked up from the skin.

RESOURCES

WEBSITES

For clinical trials currently associated with the National Institutes of Health:
   http://cancer.gov/clinicaltrials
For herbal medicine:
   www.mskcc.org/aboutherbs
Alpen Klinik: a medical model for complementary care:
   http://ursula-jacob.de
Alternative cancer therapies:
   http://cancerguide.org
Alternative medicine interactive site:
   www.alternativemedicine.com

HERBS AND SUPPLEMENTS

Health Concerns, 8001 Capwell Drive, Oakland, CA 94621 Traditional Chinese medicine herbs	800-233-9355
Dakota Providers, PO Box 8023, Fargo, ND 58109 Willard Water	800-447-4793
Symplexty Health (Cell Tech International Inc.), 565 Century Court, Klamath Falls, OR 97601	800-800-1300

Super "green" foods

Merritt Naturals, PO Box 532, Rumson, NJ 07760 Supplements for dogs and cats	888-463-7748
Biotec Foods, Honolulu, HI 96813 Enzymes	800-331-5888
Minimum Price Homeopathic Books, PO Box 2187, Blaine, WA 98231	800-663-8272
Natren, Inc., 3105 Willow Lane, Westlake Village, CA 91361 Probiotics for pets	805-371-4737
Designing Health, Inc., 28310 Avenue Crocker, Unit G, Valencia, CA 91355 The missing link	800-774-7387
Phyto-Pharmica, 825 Challenger Drive, Green Bay, WI 54311 Supplements	920-469-9099
PhysioLogics, 6565 Odell Place, Boulder, CO 80301 Supplements	800-765-6775
Tyler Encapsulations, 2204 Northwest Birdsdale, Gresham, OR 97030 Supplements	800-869-9705
Jean's Greens, 119 Sulphur Spring Road, Newport, NY 13416 Western herbs	315-845-6500
East Coast Herbs Distributor, 441 Highway 49, Wiggins, MS 39577 Chinese medicine herbs and formulas	800-283-5191
Newton Laboratories, 2360 Rockaway Industrial Boulevard, Conyers, GA 30012 Homeopathic remedies	800-448-7256
Institute for Traditional Medicine and Preventive Health Care, 2442 South East Sherman, Portland, OR 97214 Traditional Chinese medicine herb formulas: Seven Forests brand, White Tiger brand	800-544-7504

NOTES

INTRODUCTION

1. L. S. McGinnis, "Alternative Therapies, 1990: An Overview," *Cancer* 67, Supplement 6 (1991): 1788–92.

2. G. Deng and B. Cassileth, "To What Extent Do Cancer Patients Use Complementary and Alternative Medicine?" *Nature Clinical Practice Oncology* 2 (2005): 496–97.

3. G. J. Guzley, "Alternative Cancer Treatments: Impact of Unorthodox Therapy on the Patient with Cancer," *Southern Medical Journal* 85, no. 5 (1992): 519–23.

4. David M. Eisenberg et al., "Trends in Alternative Medicine Use in the United States, 1990–1999: Results of a Follow-Up National Survey," *New England Journal of Medicine* 280 (1993): 1569–75.

CHAPTER I

1. Robert Atkins, *Cancer* (Tiburon, CA: Future Medicine Publishing, 1997), 35.

2. S. P. Hauser, "Unproven Methods in Cancer Treatment," *Current Opinions in Oncology* 5, no. 4 (1993): 646–54.

3. John Boik, *Cancer and Natural Medicine* (Princeton, MN: Oregon Press, 1996), 3.

4. J. Kun, *Prevention and Treatment of Carcinoma in Traditional Chinese Medicine* (Hong Kong: The Commercial Press, 1985); M. J. Pan, Y. H. Li, and L. F. Chen, "Treatment of 120 Cases of Gastric Cancer with *li wei hua jie* Decoction Combined with Surgery and Chemotherapy," *Chinese Journal of Combined Traditional and Western Medicine* 6, no. 5 (1986): 268–70.

CHAPTER 3

1. M. Suffness, D. Newman, and K. Snader, "Discovery and Development of Antineoplastic Agents from Natural Sources," in *Bioorganic Marine Chemistry*, vol. 3 (Berlin: Springer-Verlag, 1989).

2. E. J. Park and J. M. Pezzuto, "Botanicals in Cancer Chemoprevention," *Cancer and Metastases Review* 2002: 231–55.

3. John Boik, *Cancer and Natural Medicine* (Princeton, MN: Oregon Press, 1996), 111.

CHAPTER 4

1. M. Chang, *Anticancer Medicinal Herbs* (Hunan Changsha: Human Science and Technology Press, 1992).

2. Leo Grillo, "Food Poisoning: You Are Eating California's Dead Pets," Information Sheet, October 2, 2007.

3. Joseph Farah, "Seafood Imports from China Raised in Untreated Sewage," *World News Daily*, June 4, 2007.

4. Jon Barron, *Lessons from the Miracle Doctors* (Las Vegas, NV: Healing America Inc., 2001).

5. Ruth Winter, *A Consumer's Dictionary for Food Additives* (New York: Three River Press, 2004).

CHAPTER 5

1. William Joel Meggs, *The Inflammation Cure* (New York: Contemporary Books, 2003), 47.

2. Meggs, *The Inflammation Cure*.

3. J. H. John et al., "Effects of Fruit and Vegetables Consumption on Plasma Antioxidant Concentrations and Blood Pressure: A Randomized Controlled Trial," *Lancet* 359, no. 9322 (2002): 1969–74.

4. C. P. Burns and A. A. Spector, "Effects of Lipids on Cancer Therapy," *Nutrition Review* 48, no. 6 (1990): 233–40.

5. R. Marchioli et al., "Efficacy of n-3 Poly-Unsaturated Fatty Acids after Myocardial Infarction: Results of a GISSi-Prevenzione Trial," *Lipids* 36, suppl. (2001): S119–26.

CHAPTER 6

1. John Boik, *Cancer and Natural Medicine* (Princeton, MN: Oregon Press, 1996).

2. A. M. Novi, "Regression of Aflatoxin B1-Induced Hepatocellular Carcinomas by Reduced Glutathione," *Science* 212, no. 1 (1981): 459–64.

3. Jutta Wellmann and Friedrich Dittmar, *Enzyme Therapy Basics* (New York: Sterling Publishing, 1999).

4. Jon Barron, *Lessons from the Miracle Doctors* (Las Vegas, NV: Healing America Inc., 2001), 31.

CHAPTER 7

1. MD Anderson Hospital, "High Doses of Multiple Antioxidants, Vitamins: Essential Ingredients in Improving the Efficacy of Standard Cancer Therapy," *Postgraduate Medicine* 87 (1990): 163.

2. James F. Balch, *The Super Antioxidants* (New York: Evans Company Inc., 1998).

3. John Boik, *Cancer and Natural Medicine* (Princeton, MN: Oregon Press, 1996).

4. World Cancer Research Fund and American Institute for Cancer Research, *Food, Nutrition and the Prevention of Cancer: A Global Perspective* (Washington, DC: American Institute for Cancer Research, 2007); K. N. Prasad and W. C. Cole, "Antioxidants in Cancer Therapy," *Journal of Clinical Oncology* 20, no. 24 (2000): o8–e9.

5. Balch, *The Super Antioxidants*.

6. Boik, *Cancer and Natural Medicine*.

CHAPTER 8

1. Jeanne M. Wallace, "Modulation of the Inflammatory Cascade: An Essential Target in Cancer Therapy," *International Journal of Integrative Medicine* 4, no. 5 (October/November 2002): 6–22.

2. M. Yoshida et al., "The Effects of Quercetin on Cell Cycle Progression and Growth of Human Gastric Cells," *FEBS Letters* 60 (1990): 10–13.

3. G. Kolata, "New Finding Offers Insights into How Cancer Develops, Why Tumors Resist Chemotherapy and Radiation," *New York Times*, January 4, 1996.

4. C. Yu et al., "The Progress of Treating and Preventing Cancer with Integrative Chinese and Eastern Medicine," in *Advances in Clinical Oncology*, ed. Sun Yan et al. (Beijing: Chinese Union Medical University Press, 2005), 166–82.

5. John W. Diamond and W. Lee Cowden, *Definitive Guide to Cancer* (Tiburon, CA: Future Medicine Publishing, 1997).

6. Keith I. Block, *Life over Cancer* (New York: Bantam Books, 2009).

CHAPTER 9

1. E. X. Yu et al., *The Study of Integrative Chinese and Western Medicine on Cancer Treatments* (Shanghai: Shanghai Science and Technology Press, 1985).

2. D. Abrams and Andrew Weil, *Integrative Oncology* (New York: Oxford University Press, 2009), 281; I. Bairati et al., "Antioxidant Vitamins Supplementation and Mortality:

A Randomized Trial in Head and Neck Cancer Patients," *International Journal of Cancer* 119 (2006): 2221–24.

3. Dana Ullman, "Homeopathy for Primary and Adjunctive Cancer Therapy," *Integrative Oncology* 3 (2009): 313.

CHAPTER 10

1. T. E. Rohan et al., "Dietary Fiber, Vitamins A, C, and E and the Risk of Breast Cancer: A Cohort Study," *Cancer Causes Control* 4, no. 1: 429–37.

CHAPTER 12

1. E. W. Flagg et al., "Dietary Glutathione Intake and the Risk of Oral and Pharyngeal Cancer," *American Journal of Epidemiology* 139, no. 5 (1994): 453–65; J. F. Smyth et al., "Glutathione Reduces Toxicity and Improves Quality of Life of Women Diagnosed with Ovarian Cancer Treated with Cisplatin: Results of a Double-Blind Randomized Trial," *Annals of Oncology* 8 (1997): 569–73.

2. D. T. Chu et al., "Fractionated Extract of *Astragalus membranaceus*, a Chinese Medical Herb, Potentiates LAK Cell Cytotoxicity Generated by a Low Dose of Recombinant Interleukin-2," *Journal of Clinical and Laboratory Immunology* 26, no. 4 (1988): 183–87.

3. Keith I. Block, *Life over Cancer* (New York: Bantam Books, 2009).

4. Y. Rong et al., "*Gingko biloba* Attenuates Oxidative Stress in Macrophages and Endothelial Cells," *Free Radical Biology and Medicine* 20, no. 1 (1996): 121–27.

5. D. M. Hau and Z. S. You, "Therapeutic Effects of Ginseng and Mitomycin-C on Experimental Liver Tumors," *International Journal of Oriental Medicine* 15, no. 1 (1990): 10–14.

6. John Boik, *Cancer and Natural Medicine* (Princeton, MN: Oregon Press, 1996).

7. Block, *Life over Cancer*.

8. D. Iarussi et al., "Protective Effect of Coenzyme Q10 on Cardiotoxicity," *Molecular Aspects of Medicine* 15, suppl. 1 (1994): 207–12.

9. K. Adachi et al., "Potentiation of Host-Mediated Antitumor Activity on Mice by Beta-Glucan Obtained from *Grigola frondosa*," *Chemical and Pharmacological Bulletin* 15, suppl. 1 (1987): 207–12; H. Namba, "*Maitake* Mushroom Immune Therapy to Prevent Cancer Growth and Metastasis," *Explore* 6, no. 1 (1995): 17; H. Namba, "Antitumor Activity of Orally Administered D-Fraction from *Maitake* Mushroom," *Journal of Naturopathic Medicine* 1, no. 4 (1993): 10–15.

10. H. Oka, "Protective Study of Chemoprevention of Hepatocellular Carcinoma with *Sho saiko*," *Cancer* 76, no. 5 (1995): 743–49.

CHAPTER 13

1. R. C. Yu et al., "The Progress of Treating and Preventing Cancer with Integrative Chinese and Eastern Medicine," in *Advances in Clinical Oncology*, ed. Sun Yan et al. (Beijing: Chinese Union Medical University Press, 2005), 166–82.

2. Y. Sun, *Treating and Preventing Cancer with Integrative Chinese and Western Medicine* (Beijing: Beijing Medical University and Union Medical University Press, 1995).

3. D. Z. Zhang, "A Panel Discussion on TCM's Potentiation and Attenuation Effects on Cancer Radio- and Chemotherapy," *CJITWM* 12, no. 3 (1992): 135–38.

4. H. Namba, "*Maitake* Mushroom Immune Therapy to Prevent Cancer Growth and Metastasis," *Explore* 6, no. 1 (1995): 17.

5. Dharmananda Subhuti, *Chinese Herbal Therapies for Immune Disorders* (Portland, OR: Institute for Traditional Chinese Medicine and Preventive Health Care, 1988).

6. X. Wang and C. Q. Ling, "The Progress of Anti-Metastasis Studies on Chinese Herbal Active Ingredients," *Chinese Journal of Integrated Traditional Western Medicine* 24, no. 2 (2004): 178–81.

CHAPTER 15

1. Jeanne M. Wallace, "Modulation of the Inflammatory Cascade: An Essential Target in Cancer Therapy," *International Journal of Integrative Medicine* 4, no. 5 (October/November 2002): 6–22.

2. Wallace, "Modulation of the Inflammatory Cascade."

CHAPTER 16

1. Burton Goldberg, *Alternative Medicine* (Tiburon, CA: Future Medicine Publishing, 1999), xxxv.

2. John W. Diamond and W. Lee Cowden, *Definitive Guide to Cancer* (Tiburon, CA: Future Medicine Publishing, 1997), 35.

3. Diamond and Cowden, *Definitive Guide to Cancer*.

4. Dharmananda Subhuti, *Chinese Herbal Therapies for Immune Disorders* (Portland, OR: Institute for Traditional Chinese Medicine and Preventive Health Care, 1988); W. Y. Li and E. Lien, "FuZhen Herbs in the Treatment of Cancer," *OHAI Bulletin*, no. 68 (1986): 1–8.

5. Diamond and Cowden, *Definitive Guide to Cancer*, 854.

APPENDIX A

1. John W. Diamond and W. Lee Cowden, *Definitive Guide to Cancer* (Tiburon, CA: Future Medicine Publishing, 1997).

APPENDIX C

1. John Boik, *Cancer and Natural Medicine* (Princeton, MN: Oregon Press, 1996).

APPENDIX D

1. *International Journal of Gynecological Cancer* 5 (1995): 81–86; *Cancer Chemotherapy and Pharmacology* 25 (1990): 355–60; *Tumor* 78 (1992): 374–76.

BIBLIOGRAPHY

Abrams, D., and A. Weil. *Integrative Oncology*. New York: Oxford University Press, 2009.

Adachi, K., et al. "Potentiation of Host-Mediated Antitumor Activity on Mice by Beta-Glucan Obtained from *Grigola frondosa*." *Chemical and Pharmacological Bulletin* 15, suppl. 1 (1987): 207–12.

Atkins, Robert. *Cancer*. Tiburon, CA: Future Medicine Publishing, 1997.

Bairati, I., et al. "Antioxidants, Vitamin Supplementation and Mortality: A Randomized Trial in Head and Neck Cancer Patients." *International Journal of Cancer* 119: 2221–24.

Balch, James F. *The Super Antioxidants*. New York: Evans Company Inc., 1998.

Barron, John. *Lessons from the Miracle Doctors*. Las Vegas, NV: Healing America Inc., 2001.

Block, Keith I. *Life over Cancer*. New York: Bantam Books, 2009.

Boik, John. *Cancer and Natural Medicine*. Princeton, MN: Oregon Press, 1996.

Burns, C. P., and A. A. Spector. "Effects of Lipids on Cancer Therapy." *Nutrition Review* 48, no. 6 (1990): 233–40.

Chang, M. *Anticancer Medicinal Herbs*. Hunan Changsha: Human Science and Technology Press, 1992.

Chu, D. T. et al. "Fractionated Extract of *Astragalus membranaceus*, a Chinese Medical Herb, Potentiates LAK Cell Cytotoxicity Generated by a Low Dose of Recombinant Interleukin-2." *Journal of Clinical and Laboratory Immunology* 26, no. 4 (1998): 183–87.

Deng, G., and B. Cassileth. "To What Extent Do Cancer Patients Use Complementary and Alternative Medicine?" *Nature Clinical Practice Oncology* 2, no. 10 (2005): 496–97.

Dharmananda, Subhuti. *Chinese Herbal Therapies for Immune Disorders*. Portland, OR: Institute for Traditional Chinese Medicine and Preventive Health Care, 1988.

Diamond, John W., and W. Lee Cowden. *Definitive Guide to Cancer*. Tiburon, CA: Future Medicine Publishing, 1997.

Eisenberg, David M., et al. "Trends in Alternative Medicine Use in the United States, 1990–1999: Results of a Follow-Up National Survey." *New England Journal of Medicine* 280 (1993): 1569–75.

Farar, Joseph. "Seafood Imports from China Raised in Untreated Sewage." *World News Daily*, June 4, 2007.

Gershwin, M. E., et al. "The Potential Impact of Nutritional Factors on Immunological Responsiveness." In *Nutrition and Immunity*. Orlando, FL: Academic Press, 1985.

Goldberg, Burton. *Alternative Medicine*. Tiburon, CA: Future Medicine Publishing, 1999.

Grillo, Leo. "Food Poisoning: You Are Eating California's Dead Pets." Information Sheet, October 2, 2007.

Guzley, G. J. "Alternative Cancer Treatments: Impact of Unorthodox Therapy on the Patients with Cancer." *Southern Medical Journal* 85, no. 5 (1992): 519–23.

Flagg, E. W., et al. "Dietary Glutatione Intake and the Risk of Oral and Pharyngeal Cancer." *American Journal of Epidemiology* 5 (1994): 453–65.

Hau, D. M., and Z. S. You. "Therapeutic Effects of *Ginseng* and Mitomycin-C on Experimental Liver Tumors." *International Journal of Oriental Medicine* 15, no. 1 (1996): 10–14.

Hauser, S. P. "Unproven Methods in Cancer Treatment." *Current Opinions in Oncology* 5, no. 4 (1993): 646–54.

Iarussi, D., et al. "Protective Effect of Coenzyme Q10 on Cardiotoxicity." *Molecular Aspects of Medicine* 15, suppl. 1 (1994): 207–12.

John, J. H., et al. "Effects of Fruit and Vegetables Consumption on Plasma Antioxidant Concentrations and Blood Pressure: A Randomized Controlled Trial." *Lancet* 359, no. 9322 (2002): 1969–74.

Kantor, A. F., et al. "Urinary Tract Infections and Risk of Bladder Cancer." *American Journal of Epidemiology* 119, no. 40 (1984): 510–15.

Kolata, G. "New Finding Offers Insight into How Cancer Develops: Why Tumors Resist Chemotherapy and Radiation." *New York Times*, June 4, 1996.

Kun, J. *Prevention and Treatment of Carcinoma in Traditional Chinese Medicine*. Hong Kong: The Commercial Press, 1985.

Li, W. Y., and E. Lien. "FuZhen Herbs in the Treatment of Cancer." *OHAI Bulletin*, no. 68 (1986), 1–8.

Marchioli, R., et al. "Efficacy of n-3 Poly-Unsaturated Fatty Acids after Myocardial Infarction: Results of a GISSi-Prevenzione Trial." *Lipids* 36, suppl. (2001): S119–26.

McGinnis, L. S. "Alternative Therapies, 1990: An Overview." *Cancer* 67, suppl. 6 (1991): 1788–92.

Meggs, William Joel. *The Inflammation Cure*. New York: Contemporary Books, 2003.

Messina, M., and S. Barnes. "The Role of Soy Products in Reducing Risk of Cancer." *Journal of the National Cancer Institute* 83, no. 8 (1991): 541–46.

Namba, H. "Antitumor Activity of Orally Administered D-Fraction from *Maitake* Mushroom." *Journal of Naturopathic Medicine* 1, no. 4 (1993): 10–15.

Namba, H. "*Maitake* Mushroom Immune Therapy to Prevent Cancer Growth and Metastasis." *Explore* 6, no. 1 (1995): 17.

Nogabhushan, M., and S. V. Bhide. "Curcumin as an Inhibitor of Cancer." *Journal of the American College of Nutrition* 11, no. 2 (1992): 192–98.

Novi, A. M. "Regression of Aflatoxin B1-Induced Hepatocellular Carcinomas by Reduced Glutathione." *Science* 212, no. 1 (1981): 459–64.

Oka, H. "Protective Study of Chemoprevention of Hepatocellular Carcinoma with *Sho saiko*." *Cancer* 76, no. 5 (1995): 743–49.

Pan, M. J., Y. H. Li, and L. F. Chen. "Treatment of 120 Cases of Gastric Cancer with *li wei hua jie* Decoction Combined with Surgery and Chemotherapy." *Chinese Journal of Combined Traditional and Western Medicine* 6, no. 5 (1986): 268–70.

Park, F. J., and J. M. Pezzuto. "Botanical Chemoprevention." *Cancer and Metastases Review* 2002: 231–55.

Prasad, K. N., and W. C. Cole. "Antioxidants in Cancer Therapy." *Journal of Clinical Oncology* 20, no. 24 (2006): e8–e9.

Reich, R., et al. "Eicosapentaenoic Acid Reduces the Invasive and Metastatic Activity of Malignant Tumor Cells." *Biochemical and Biophysical Research Communications* 160, no. 2 (1989): 59–65.

Rohan, T. E., et al. "Dietary Fiber, Vitamins A, C, and E and the Risk of Breast Cancer: A Cohort Study." *Cancer Causes Control* 4, no. 1 (1993): 29–37.

Rong, Y., et al. "*Ginkgo biloba* Attenuates Oxidative Stress in Macrophages and Endothelial Cells." *Free Radical Biology and Medicine* 20, no. 1 (1996): 121–27.

Shacter Weitzman, S. "Chronic Inflammation and Cancer." *Oncology* 16, no. 2 (2002): 217–32.

Smyth, J. F., et al. "Glutathione Reduces Toxicity and Improves Quality of Life of Women Diagnosed with Ovarian Cancer Treated with Cisplatin: Results of a Double-Blind Randomized Trial." *Annals of Oncology* 8 (1997): 569–73.

Suffness, M., D. Newman, and K. Snader. "Discovery and Development of Antineoplastic Agents from Natural Sources." In *Bioorganic Marine Chemistry*, vol. 3. Berlin: Springer-Verlag, 1989.

Sun, Y. *Treating and Preventing Cancer with Integrative Chinese and Western Medicine.* Beijing: Beijing Medical University and Union Medical University Press, 1995.

Ullman, Dana. "Homeopathy for Primary and Adjunctive Cancer Therapy." *Integrative Oncology* 3 (2009): 313.

Wallace, Jeanne M. "Modulation of the Inflammatory Cascade: An Essential Target in Cancer Therapy." *International Journal of Integrative Medicine* 4, no. 5 (October/November 2002): 6–22.

Wellmann, Jutta, and Friedrich Dittmar. *Enzyme Therapy Basics.* New York: Sterling Publishing, 1999.

Winter, Ruth. *A Consumer's Dictionary for Food Additives.* New York: Three River Press, 2004.

World Cancer Research Fund and American Institute for Cancer Research. *Food Nutrition and the Prevention of Cancer: A Global Perspective.* Washington, DC: American Institute for Cancer Research, 2007.

Yamamoto, I., et al. "Antitumor Effect of Seaweeds." *Japanese Journal of Experimental Medicine* 44 (1974): 543–46.

Yoshida, M., et al. "The Effects of Quercetin on Cell Cycle Progression and Growth of Human Gastric Cells." *FEBS Letters* 60 (1990): 10–13.

Yu, E. X., et al. *The Study of Integrative Chinese and Western Medicine on Cancer Treatment*. Shanghai: Shanghai Science and Technology Press, 1985.

Yu, R. C., et al. "The Progress of Treating and Preventing Cancer with Integrative Chinese and Eastern Medicine." In *Advances in Clinical Oncology*, edited by Sun Yan et al. Beijing: Chinese Union Medical University Press, 2005, 166–82.

Zhang, D. Z. "A Panel Discussion on TCM's Potentiation and Attenuation Effects on Cancer Radio- and Chemotherapy." *CJITWM* 12, no. 3 (1992): 135.

INDEX

ABOUT THE AUTHOR

Marie Cargill is a licensed acupuncturist, registered herbalist and homeopath, and member of the American Association of Oriental Medicine. She has thirty-five years of experience in the field of alternative medicine and was the first practitioner of alternative animal care—acupuncture and herbal medicine—in New England. Cargill has been featured in *Time* Magazine, *The Boston Globe*, *The Boston Herald*, *National Geographic*, and *Prevention*. She has also written several other books on alternative and holistic medicine.